The Hand

This book is dedicated to our families

Kevin, Nina, my mother Hildegard and father Erwin
David, Annika and Julia
Joyce, John, Christine and Bruce

The Hand

Fundamentals of therapy
Second edition

Judith Boscheinen-Morrin, MAAOT
Hand Therapist, Sydney Hospital Hand Unit, Sydney, Australia;
Founding Member of the Australian Hand Therapy Association

Victoria Davey, MCSP, MAPA
Hand Therapist, formerly of Sydney Hospital Physiotherapy
Department, Sydney, Australia

W. Bruce Conolly, FRCS, FRACS, FACS
Associate Professor of Hand Surgery, University of New South Wales;
Director of Sydney Hospital Hand Unit, Sydney, Australia

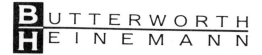

Butterworth-Heinemann
Linacre House, Jordan Hill, Oxford OX2 8DP
A division of Reed Educational and Professional Publishing Ltd

◯ A member of the Reed Elsevier plc group

OXFORD   BOSTON   JOHANNESBURG
MELBOURNE   NEW DELHI   SINGAPORE

First published 1895
Reprinted 1987, 1990
Second edition 1992
Reprinted 1995, 1997

British Library Cataloguing in Publication Data
A catalogue record for this book is available from the British Library

Library of Congress Cataloguing in Publication Data
A catalogue record for this book is available from the Library of Congress

ISBN 0 7506 0570 7

Printed and bound in Great Britain by Hartnolls Ltd, Bodmin, Cornwall

Contents

Preface

There is no doubt that the surgical and therapeutic management of hand injuries and conditions has become a specialized area of medicine and therapy. Despite this trend, however, many hand patients will find themselves in the care of doctors and therapists who are responsible for the management of a great variety of conditions, hand problems representing only a small percentage of their caseload.

The purpose of this book is to provide an easy reference and treatment guide for those whose experience with hand patients is limited. We wish to highlight the common complications associated with specific injuries and illustrate how these can be overcome.

We have confined our text to the discussion of the more commonly encountered hand conditions and therefore omit sections such as prosthetic training. Also, for the sake of brevity, very detailed anatomy, functional anatomy and methods of muscle testing are not included in this book as there are many excellent texts to which the reader can refer.

While discussion of pain syndromes in general is not included, a short chapter on reflex sympathetic dystrophy has been added. This condition, although not an everyday complication, can wreak havoc on the hand and upper limb if not recognized and promptly treated in its earliest stages.

Acknowledgements

The authors wish to express their sincere thanks to:

Kevin Morrin, for embellishment of the text through additional artwork.

Anne Smidlin, Head of Sydney Hospital Occupational Therapy Department, for continuing support and encouragement.

Eveline Gallard, Hand Unit secretary, for assistance with camera work.

Joanne Munro, Senior Hand Therapist, Sydney Hospital Physiotherapy Department, for acting as a professional 'sounding board'.

Hope Kennedy and Louise Cutts, personal secretaries to Professor W. Bruce Conolly, for their kind patience during photocopying sessions.

The many patients who cooperated so willingly during photographic sessions.

Abbreviations

Joints

DIP   Distal interphalangeal
IP   Interphalangeal
MCP   Metacarpophalangeal
PIP   Proximal interphalangeal
CMC   Carpometacarpal

Muscles and tendons

ADM   Abductor digiti minimi (or quinti)
APB   Abductor pollicis brevis
APL   Abductor pollicis longus
ECRB   Extensor carpi radialis brevis
ECRL   Extensor carpi radialis longus
ECU   Extensor carpi ulnaris
EDC   Extensor digitorum communis
EDM   Extensor digiti minimi (or quinti)
EI   Extensor indicis (or proprius)
EPB   Extensor pollicis brevis
EPL   Extensor pollicis longus
FCR   Flexor carpi radialis
FCU   Flexor carpi ulnaris
FDM   Flexor digiti minimi
FDP   Flexor digitorum profundus
FDS   Flexor digitorum superficialis (or sublimis)
FPL   Flexor pollicis longus
ODM   Opponens digiti minimi
PL   Palmaris longus
PT   Pronator teres

Miscellaneous

ADL	Activities of daily living
POSI	Position of safe immobilization
RSD	Reflex sympathetic dystrophy
TENS	Transcutaneous electrical nerve stimulation

Introduction

Effective hand therapy assumes:

1 An understanding of functional hand anatomy.
2 A team approach with regular liaison among team members.

The patient is the most important member of this team and his education and co-operation with treatment are the basis for a successful result.

The commonest problems encountered in treatment are pain, swelling and stiffness. Their prompt and correct management is vital if proper hand function is to be restored.

The mainstays of hand therapy are:

1 Oedema control.
2 Exercise.
3 Scar management.
4 Splintage.
5 Functional activity.

Wound healing

Hand therapy techniques are based on the principles of wound healing. It is important for the therapist to understand these principles in order to formulate a safe and appropriate treatment programme (Tables 0.1 and 0.2).

Oedema

Tissue trauma disrupts capillary integrity. The blood and serum

Table 0.1 *Phases of wound healing*

Phase	Onset	Peak	Duration	Pathophysiology	Wound strength	Management
Traumatic inflammation	0	12 h	24–48 h	Vascular response; bleeding, oedema Cellular (phagocytosis) response: leucocytes, macrophages	Negligible	Rest Elevation Ice
Proliferation of fibroblasts	12 h	2–5 days	10 days	Fibroblasts proliferate, migrate and bridge wound edges by 5 days	Some	Rest Elevation
Collagen (fibroplasia)	5 days	3 months	6 months	Collagen fibrils: initially weak random fibrils, later strong flexible fibres depending on the stress placed upon them	Rapid rise	Splintage of the repaired tissue Exercise
Remodelling	1 month	→	2 years plus	Collagenase removes excess collagen, fibroblasts contract, and there is vascular and wound shrinkage	Continued gradual rise	Exercise and return of function

Table 0.2 *Healing table*

Tissue	Early healing (movement without stress) (weeks)	Consolidated healing (can take full stress) (weeks)
Skin	1	3
Tendon to tendon	3	6–12
Tendon to bone	3	6–12
Ligament repair	As for tendon	As for tendon
Nerve	3	6
Bone to bone	3	6–12

These healing times vary according to the age, local blood supply and general condition of the patient.

that leaks from damaged vessels into surrounding tissue is termed oedema.

The supply of blood to the arm and hand is dependent on the arterial pressure. The arterial system of the forearm and hand is situated volarly while the return pathways, i.e. the veins and lymphatics, are situated dorsally.

The return flow through the veins and lymphatics is dependent on the pumping mechanism which is brought about by the active movements of the arm and hand. When this mechanism is compromised by injury and/or immobilization, there is poor fluid return and hence a tendency for oedema to remain unresolved.

The swollen hand will assume a 'claw' position (Figure 0.1) in which the metacarpophalangeal (MCP) joints are placed into extension while the interphalangeal (IP) joints assume a flexed position.

The various tissues, i.e. tendons, nerves, vessels, joints and intrinsic musculature are compromised by reduced nutrition and become fibrosed. The greater the oedema and the longer it persists, the more extensive the resultant fibrosis will be.

Position of safe immobilization

Correct positioning of the hand following injury is most important. Unless contraindicated, e.g. after nerve or tendon repair, the

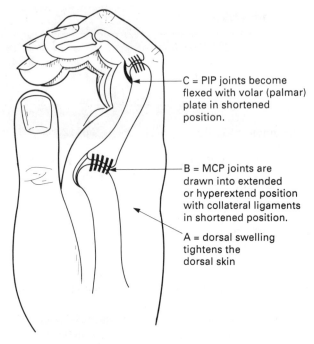

C = PIP joints become flexed with volar (palmar) plate in shortened position.

B = MCP joints are drawn into extended or hyperextend position with collateral ligaments in shortened position.

A = dorsal swelling tightens the dorsal skin

Figure 0.1   *Oedema on the dorsum of the hand places the MCP joints in extension while the IP joints assume a flexed position*

hand is placed as closely as possible to the position of safe immobilization (POSI).

This position is as follows:

1 Wrist in 30–40 degrees extension.
2 MCP joints in maximum flexion.
3 IP joints in maximum extension.
4 Thumb in palmar abduction, the pulp of the thumb being in line with the pulps of the index and middle fingers (Figure 0.2).

In this position, the collateral ligaments of the MCP joints and the volar plates of the IP joints are fully stretched, thereby preventing extension contractures of the MCP joints or flexion contractures of the IP joints respectively (Figure 0.3). Because the thumb is positioned to keep the first web space open, an adduction contracture of the thumb is also prevented.

In response to the changing status of the oedema, a number of

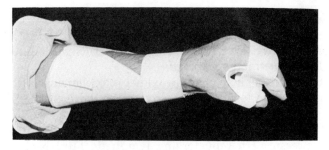

Figure 0.2 *Position of safe immobilization*

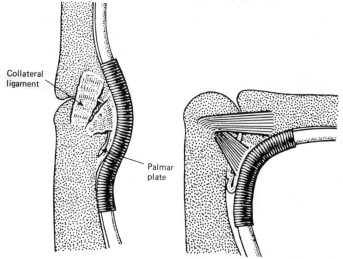

Collateral
ligament

Palmar
plate

Figure 0.3 *Collateral ligaments of the MCP joints are relaxed and short when the joints are extended, and stretched when the joints are flexed*

modifications to the original splint may be necessary before the desired position is achieved.

Oedema control

Prompt management of oedema is mandatory if the ensuing fibrosis of unresolved oedema is to be avoided.

Oedema is effectively managed in the following ways:

1 Constant high elevation: effective elevation means that the hand is positioned above the elbow and the elbow above the shoulder.

2 Cold therapy: cold therapy reduces oedema by causing a vasoconstriction of the capillaries. When applying ice packs, a thin dressing layer will prevent ice burn while allowing the cold to penetrate to the tissues.

Small areas such as the proximal interphalangeal (PIP) joint can be treated locally with an ice cube or with crushed ice held in a cloth.

3 Intermittent pressure: intermittent pressure increases interstitial pressure, thereby forcing lymphatic fluid back into the venous system.

To be effective, the pressure must be greater than the capillary pressure, i.e. 25 mmHg. The arm is elevated on pillows and the pressure regulated in accordance with each patient's tolerance and condition. Treatment times vary from 15 min to 2 h (Figure 0.4).

4 Retrograde massage: retrograde massage is another effective modality for dispersing oedema. Massage should begin distally and progress proximally.

5 Active movement: when permitted, the patient should be encouraged to move all fingers actively in an effort to form a fist. The hand should be in elevation and exercises should be performed in a methodical and sustained manner; merely wriggling the fingers will not be effective. Active flexion should be followed by efforts to achieve maximum extension.

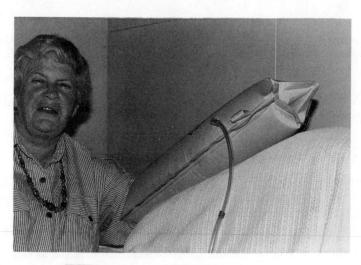

Figure 0.4   *Intermittent pressure treatment*

While some discomfort is acceptable, exercise should not cause pain. Over-vigorous exercise will not only cause pain which often results in loss of the patient's confidence, but also perpetuates the pain-swelling-stiffness cycle.

In conjunction with attendance at formal therapy sessions, a suitable home programme is prescribed for each patient. This programme should be carried out 1–2 hourly; without this continuity, the therapist's efforts will be futile.

Following injury and/or immobilization of the hand, it is important to maintain the mobility of all upper limb joints.

6 Compression measures: a Lycra glove, Lycra finger stall, Coban wrap (2.5 or 5 cm), Tubigrip (usually sizes C, D and E) and string wrapping are effective means of reducing oedema and maintaining this reduction (Figures 0.5 and 0.6).

Isotoner gloves can be purchased from most department stores or medical suppliers. Gloves are worn inside-out to prevent discomfort from seams. They can be worn during exercise/activity and at night.

Coban wrap (5 cm) can be used for acute hand oedema where application of a glove may be impossible or impractical.

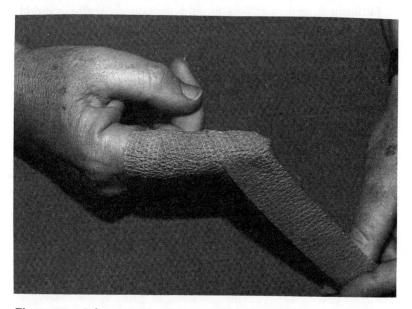

Figure 0.5 *Coban wrap is a comfortable and effective means of reducing oedema without restricting movement*

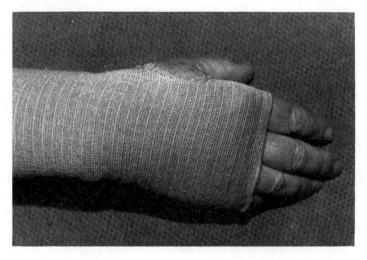

Figure 0.6   *Tubigrip (single or double layer) provides even compression for effective oedema reduction at wrist and forearm level as well as on the dorsum of the hand*

Tubigrip stocking can be applied with either a single or double layer.

Digital oedema is managed with a Lycra finger stall which is easily made, or 2.5 cm Coban which is applied distally to proximally with even pressure; these can be worn continuously.

String wrapping, like 2.5 cm Coban, is applied in a distal-to-proximal direction and is left in place for approximately 5 min. A soft cotton cord of several millimetres thickness is most suitable. On removal of the string, the patient performs active flexion/extension exercises to capitalize on oedema reduction (Figure 0.7).

With any of these above measures, the degree of pressure should be compatible with comfort and should not result in numbness, throbbing or discoloration of the hand or digit. These measures are contraindicated where oedema is due to inflammation or infection.

Scar management

Scar formation is a normal biological process necessary for healing; however, successful wound healing is not always synonymous with smooth tendon glide and good function.

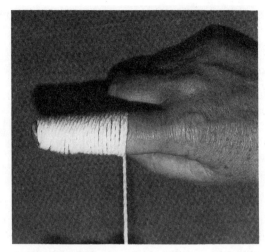

Figure 0.7   *String wrapping of individual digits is effective in oedema reduction before exercise sessions*

Because in the hand so many structures co-exist in a confined space, it is inevitable that these various structures will become adherent to one another during the healing process, e.g. skin-tendon-bone adhesion following extensor tendon repair on the dorsum of the hand.

Scar tissue formation will be adversely affected by such factors as unresolved oedema, haematoma or infection.

While rest is indicated in the inflammatory phase of wound healing, active exercise is instituted during the fibroplastic and remodelling phases.

Scar tissue formed during fibroplasia is a dense structure of randomly oriented collagen fibres. During the remodelling phase there is a change in the weave of these fibres into a more organized pattern. This pattern can be influenced by applying physical forces such as tension and stress. This can be achieved by means of: massage, compression (pressure), stretching and electrical therapy (ultrasound).

Massage

Massage applies compressive and distractive forces directly to the scar which helps loosen underlying tissues which may have become adherent, e.g. following multiple flexor tendon repair at the wrist.

Compression

Compression can be achieved by way of a Lycra finger stall or glove, Coban wrap, Tubigrip stocking and various silicone moulds, e.g. Silicone elastomer, Otoform-K, gelsheet. The moulds can be held in place by a bandage or by a glove or Tubigrip stocking where appropriate (Figure 0.8).

Stretching

Stretch is a passive action which results in elongation of the elastic elements of various tissues. This can be achieved by manual stretching, active exercises and splinting. Splinting should provide a gentle continuous force rather than an intense intermittent one.

Electrical therapy (ultrasound)

Ultrasound has been shown to cause changes in the patterning of

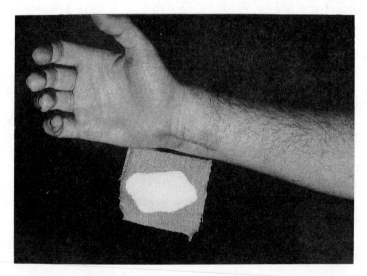

Figure 0.8   *Silicone elastomer moulds or gel sheet can be used under the pressure of a Lycra glove or Tubigrip stocking*

collagen fibres as well as increasing circulation. It is thought that this change in patterning may help in the remodelling and softening of scar tissue.

Splintage

See Chapter 15.
A splint may be prescribed for any of the following reasons:

1 Immobilization following surgery or injury.
2 Support, protection or rest, e.g. the acute rheumatoid hand, carpal tunnel syndrome or De Quervain's syndrome.
3 To prevent deformity, e.g. a 'spaghetti' splint to prevent a 'claw' deformity following an ulnar nerve injury.
4 To correct a joint or soft tissue contracture, e.g. a dynamic MCP flexion splint for an MCP extension contracture.

Splints must be used judiciously and should:

1 Fulfil the purpose for which they are prescribed.
2 Fit accurately and comfortably and be aesthetically acceptable to the patient.
3 Be reviewed on a regular basis to assess efficacy.
4 Where appropriate, be removed regularly throughout the day so that all splinted joints are fully exercised.
5 Be discarded when no longer effective.

Functional activity

The patient should be encouraged to use the hand normally as soon as it is considered safe to do so. Light, non-resistive selfcare activities can usually be commenced within a few weeks or often days of injury and do much to instil confidence and hasten the restoration of hand function.

1

Assessment

Clinical Assessment

History taking

The patient is asked about the time and the nature of onset of the disorder. In the case of trauma, the patient is asked about the mechanism of injury and the details, if any, of previous treatment.

Visual

Look for:

1 Wounds.
2 Circulation: this is indicated by colour, which may be pale, red or cyanosed.
3 Skin condition: excessive dryness is a feature of nerve damage. A tight (diminished skin creases) and/or shiny appearance may be a sign of reflex sympathetic dystrophy (RSD): excessive sweating (hyperhidrosis) can also be indicative of RSD.
4 Oedema.
5 Deformity.
6 Muscle wasting.
7 Condition of the nails (e.g. brittle), hair (e.g. coarse) and pulps of the fingers (e.g. wasting, 'pencil-point' appearance).

A simple hand diagram depicting the palm and/or dorsum can be used to record oedema, sensory impairment, scarring, neuroma site or amputation (Figure 1.1).

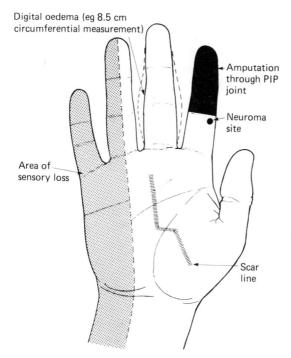

Digital oedema (eg 8.5 cm circumferential measurement)

Amputation through PIP joint

Neuroma site

Area of sensory loss

Scar line

Figure 1.1 *Simple line drawing of the hand used to illustrate loss of sensation, scar line, neuroma or oedema*

Tactile

Assess by touch:

1 Temperature: increased temperature may indicate infection, decreased temperature may be a sign of poor circulation or nerve injury.
2 Scar condition: for instance, mobile or adherent, or hypertrophic or flat.
3 Hypersensitivity: this may indicate a neuroma.
4 Excessive sweating or dryness of the skin.
5 Joint or soft tissue tightness.

Pain

The patient is asked to describe the nature of the pain experienced, e.g. stabbing, shooting, burning or aching.

The level of pain experienced by the patient may be graded on a scale of one to ten, with ten representing the severest degree of pain. This level is assessed before and after each treatment where appropriate and can be represented on a pain chart (Figure 1.2).

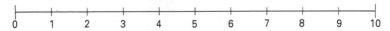

Figure 1.2   *Pain chart on which the patient can indicate his degree of pain before and after treatment*

During any examination or treatment, the hand should always be moved gently and slowly. If initial handling results in pain, there will result a fear of treatment and loss of confidence; this is especially true of young children and the elderly.

Range of movement

As soon as the immediate post-traumatic/surgical phase is over, the passive and/or active range of movement is recorded using a small goniometer. For consistency, these movements should ideally be measured each time by the same therapist.

It is important to ensure that the more proximal joints, that is the elbow and wrist, are held in a constant position: if the wrist is flexed, IP flexion will be limited; conversely, if the wrist is overextended then finger extension will be limited.

The measurements are taken with the forearm supported on a table in the midposition and the wrist in 30–40 degrees extension.

Range of movement is usually expressed as extension/flexion with 0 degrees regarded as neutral (Figures 1.3 and 1.4).

For example, 20/105 active movement of the PIP joint of the right index finger denotes a 20 degree extension lag (or flexion deformity) and a limit of 105 degrees flexion. In other words, there is an active range of 85 degrees of joint movement.

To gain an impression of digital joint movement, the distance from the pulp of the finger to the midpalm is noted (Figure 1.5). This method is not as accurate as using a goniometer because the MCP joint is not always in a constant position.

Thumb web span in both the extended and abducted positions should also be assessed by measuring with a ruler the distance between the tips of the thumb and of the index finger.

Oedema

Oedema can be assessed by using a tape measure at the base of the fingers, around the PIP joints and at the level of the MCP joints (Figure 1.6).

Another method of measuring oedema is by means of water

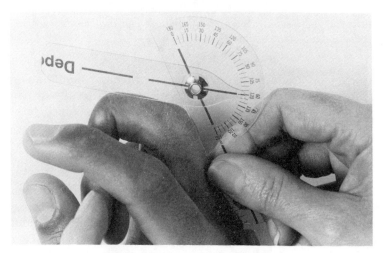

Figure 1.3   *Active PIP flexion range of the middle finger is measured with a small goniometer*

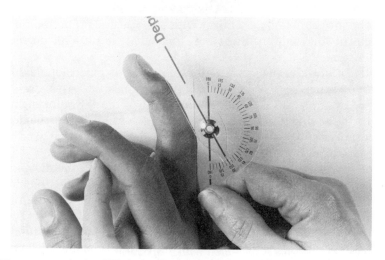

Figure 1.4   *Active PIP extension range of the middle finger is recorded*

displacement when the hand is immersed in a large container, such as a Perspex tank, with markings indicating the volume. The tank is filled to a known level and the hand and wrist are held vertically and placed into the tank to a predetermined level

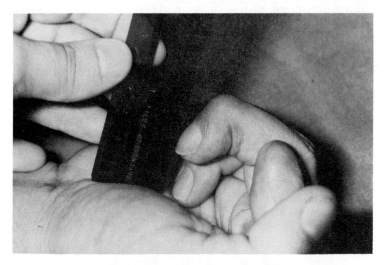

Figure 1.5   *Impression of digital flexion can be gained by measuring the distance from the fingertip to the midpalm*

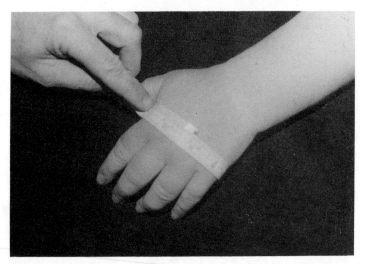

Figure 1.6   *Oedema is measured with a tape measure at the level of the MCP joints and a comparison is made with the unaffected hand*

marked circumferentially on the forearm. When the water settles after rising, the difference in volume is recorded. A comparison is then made with the non-involved extremity, bearing in mind that the right hand of a right-handed person will displace 15–20 ml more than the non-dominant hand.

Sensation

The aims of sensory assessment are:

1 To determine the extent of sensory loss.
2 To assist in the diagnosis of neuropathies, compression syndromes (e.g. carpal tunnel syndrome) and peripheral nerve lesions.
3 To monitor sensory recovery following nerve repair.
4 For medico-legal purposes.
5 To determine when sensory re-education should commence.
6 To determine the degree of functional impairment.

The sensory areas of the hand that are supplied by the median, ulnar and radial nerves are shown in Figures 1.7–1.9.

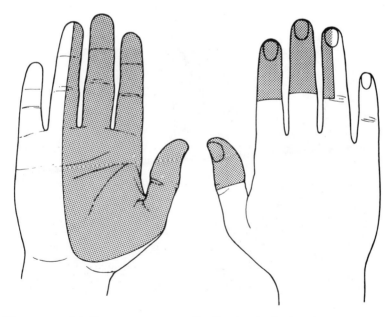

Figure 1.7 *Median nerve sensory distribution in the hand*

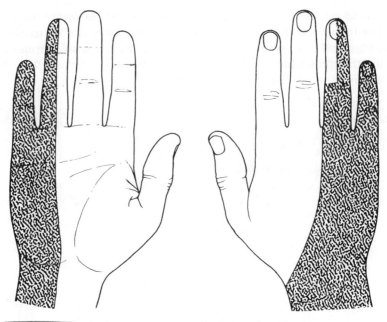

Figure 1.8 *Ulnar nerve sensory distribution in the hand*

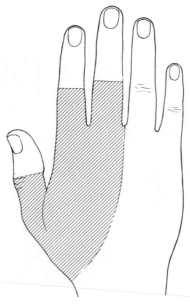

Figure 1.9 *Radial nerve sensory distribution in the hand*

If nerve injury is present, the following sensory modalities should be recorded diagrammatically and dated for follow-up assessment. (To ensure reliability and accuracy of response, stimuli are applied in an unpredictable pattern with variation in timing.)

1 Intact: quick and accurate response.
2 Absent: no response.
3 Impaired: delayed response, variable accuracy of response, or a sensation inappropriate to the stimulus, such as deep pressure perceived as a light touch.

Methods of stimulation are given below.

Light touch

Cotton wool is applied lightly to an area of the skin and the patient indicates where contact is perceived.

Pressure

Firm pressure is applied using a fingertip. The pressure should be sufficiently firm to stimulate the deep receptors without causing joint movement.

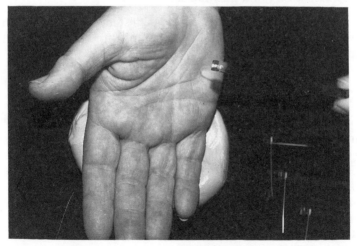

Figure 1.10   *Testing with monofilaments to assess light touch and deep pressure*

The Semmes–Weinstein test using monofilaments can be a reliable and accurate method of assessing light touch and deep pressure. Standard application of the stimuli and regular calibration of the monofilaments are necessary for maintaining objectivity of the test (Figure 1.10).

The testing set consists of 20 graded monofilaments which are precisely calibrated and of equal length. There is also a set of five monofilaments which will test the highest calculated force of each sensory level, i.e. normal, diminished light touch, diminished protective sensation, loss of protective sensation and untestable (Figure 1.11).

Pain

A pin is applied perpendicularly and at a constant pressure. To verify the accuracy of the response, a pin with a sharp and a blunt end is used so that random testing can be carried out.

Temperature

Capped test tubes filled with hot or cold water can be used for this test.

Proprioception (joint position sense)

To reduce tactile input, the part to be tested is held laterally and each joint is moved several times in all directions. The patient imitates the movement with the other hand.

Two-point discrimination (static)

The two-point discrimination (2PD) test is regarded as a test of functional sensibility because it relates to the ability of the hand to carry out fine tasks (Table 1.1).

Two compass points are applied simultaneously to an area of the skin and the distance between them is gradually decreased to determine how closely they can be brought together before the stimulus is perceived as one point.

Comparable areas on the unaffected hand should be tested because 2PD varies slightly from person to person and may vary with different occupations.

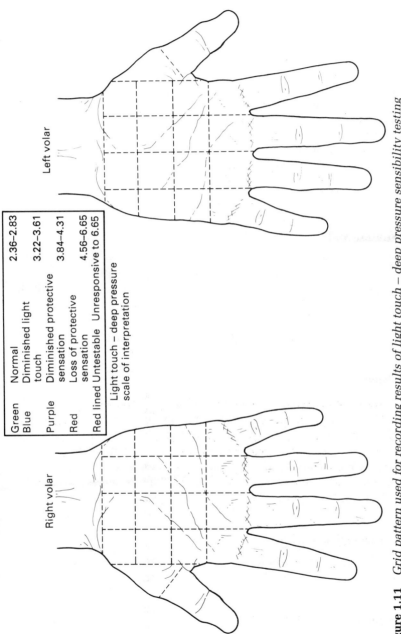

Figure 1.11 *Grid pattern used for recording results of light touch – deep pressure sensibility testing*

Left volar

Right volar

Green	Normal	2.36–2.83
Blue	Diminished light touch	3.22–3.61
Purple	Diminished protective sensation	3.84–4.31
Red	Loss of protective sensation	4.56–6.65
Red lined	Untestable	Unresponsive to 6.65

Light touch – deep pressure
scale of interpretation

Table 1.1   *Two-point discrimination in the hand*

	Distance (mm)
Pulp of the thumb	2.5–5
Pulp of the index finger	3–5
Pulp of the other digits	4–5
Base of the palmar aspect of the digits	5–6
Thenar and hypothenar eminences	5–9
Midpalmar region	11
Dorsal aspect of the digits	6–9
Dorsal aspect of the hand	7–12

After Tubiana, 1984.

Stereognosis

This is most appropriate to median nerve involvement. With vision occluded the patient is asked to identify a variety of everyday objects, beginning with larger objects such as a matchbox and a cake of soap and progressing to smaller objects such as a coin, a key and a safety pin.

Slowness or inaccuracy of response is recorded.

Tinel's sign

Tinel's sign can give an indication of the level of sensory nerve regeneration; this indication is not infallible. To test for this sign the examiner taps along the course of the nerve in a distal to proximal direction. The point at which the patient experiences paraesthesia (pins and needles) is regarded as the level to which sensory regeneration has occurred. This is called a positive Tinel's sign.

Abnormal sensations

Any abnormal sensations are noted, e.g. hypersensitivity and paraesthesia (pins and needles).

Manual muscle testing

Manual muscle testing is useful in:

1 Helping to monitor nerve regeneration
2 Preoperative evaluation of potential muscles for tendon transfer.

Grading of strength is as follows:

0 No evidence of contraction.
1 Evidence of slight muscle contraction, no joint movement.
2 Muscle contraction producing movement with gravity eliminated.
3 Muscle contraction producing movement against gravity.
4 Muscle contraction producing movement against gravity with some resistance.
5 Muscle contraction producing movement against full resistance.

Grip strength

The normal functions of the hand involve power grip and precision handling.

Power grip is primarily a function of the ulnar side of the hand (Figure 1.12).

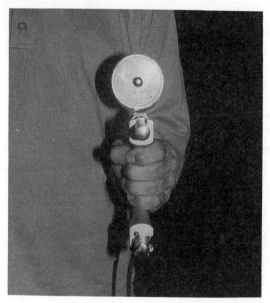

Figure 1.12 *Power grip strength is reliably measured by a Jamar grip dynamometer*

Precision handling involves the radial side of the hand where fine manipulative movements are carried out between the thumb and the tips of the index and middle fingers (Figure 1.13).

When testing the various grip strengths, comparison should be made with the unaffected side rather than with other patients, as the normal value varies considerably with age and occupation.

Dominance must be considered when making comparisons.

The tests are repeated three times, a short interval being allowed in between tests; the average reading is then recorded.

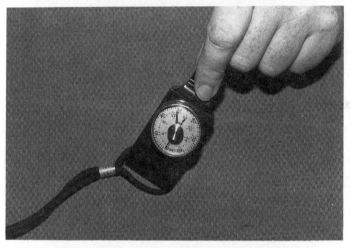

Figure 1.13   *Pincer grip function is assessed using a pinch grip meter*

Functional assessment

The patient is assessed for any problems in carrying out activities of daily living (ADL). Aids can be provided temporarily to encourage early function, e.g. built-up handles on utensils such as cutlery or razor, in the early postinjury or postoperative stage (Figure 1.14).

Complex injuries or conditions such as rheumatoid disease require full functional assessments of all aspects of the patient's daily life, that is home, work and leisure activities. These assessments may need to be carried out at regular intervals in accordance with progress or, as with the rheumatoid hand, following an exacerbation of the condition.

A home or work visit may be indicated if permanent modifica-

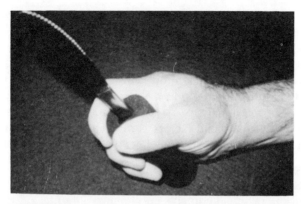

Figure 1.14 *Rubber insulation tubing can be used to build up small handles of everyday utensils*

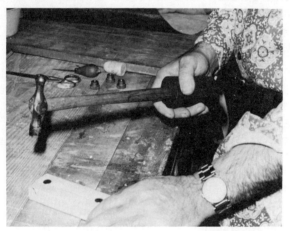

Figure 1.15 *Following severe laceration of all finger flexor tendons with skeletal damage, this 55-year-old right-handed carpenter required modification of his work tools*

tions to tools of a trade or the home environment are necessary (Figure 1.15).

Psychosocial assessment

The psychological implications of hand injuries are many in number and complex in nature. To some patients, disturbance of body image and loss of self-esteem are of major consequence; to others the potential loss of function is more important.

An individual's reaction to injury is not always proportional to the extent of the physical damage to the hand. Insight into the cultural and religious background of a patient can often provide important clues which help in management, especially in understanding reaction to pain.

Consideration of social factors is also very important. There is likely to be:

1 Disruption of family life.
2 Temporary or permanent loss of employment.
3 Disruption of social contacts and leisure pursuits.

Maintenance of motivation is vital in what might be a long-term treatment programme. Motivation can be assessed in terms of how cooperative the patient is and to what extent he utilizes his own physical and psychological resources to help himself. Motivation can be influenced by many factors including:

1 Actual degree of injury and how this threatens work and leisure activities.
2 Support provided by family and friends.
3 Any personal problems before the injury.
4 Opportunities for the patient to take a vital role in the decision-making process.
5 Level of intelligence of the patient.
6 Any language difficulties.

Prolonged hospitalization may be indicated to ensure that there is adequate supervision for those patients who have limited understanding of what is expected of them.

Interpreter services should be fully utilized and family support and participation encouraged to maintain the patient's morale.

Reactions to trauma and disease may include:

1 Fear.
2 Anxiety.
3 Withdrawal.
4 Depression.
5 Anger.
6 Dependency.
7 Mourning.

Jenny Chvala Spegal

Sorry we didnt have

a change to see

each other! Take

care + good luck on

boards + keep in

touch!

Jenn
"Wolffie"

ire can usually be
uch information as
involved.

n maintaining the
therapist must be
nd to answer the

n achievable goals
eedback when they

dealt with by the
e reactions such as
e best handled by
t of psychological
st, or psychiatrist.
e reactions hinder

pects of hand injury.

(eds) (1990) *Rehabili-
edn, C. V. Mosby, St.

nplications*, 2nd edn,

of hand injuries. In
(eds. J. M. Hunter, L.
Mosby, St. Louis, pp.

uries: A Therapeutic
. 15–59
function in the hand.

Tubiana, R. (1984) *Examination of the Hand and Upper Limb*, W. B. Saunders, Philadelphia

2

Flexor tendons

Anatomy

Flexor tendons are thick white cords of specialized fibrous tissue that transmit muscle action across joints. The tendons are restrained by annular and cruciate ligaments (or pulleys) at the wrist and in the digits (Figure 2.1).

The annular and cruciate ligaments improve the mechanical efficiency of tendon excursion by preventing bowstringing. The annular ligaments are thick and rigid, while the cruciate ligaments which lie over the joints are thin and flexible to allow movement.

The A2 and A4 pulleys are the most important ones to repair or reconstruct after injury to prevent bowstringing of the tendon.

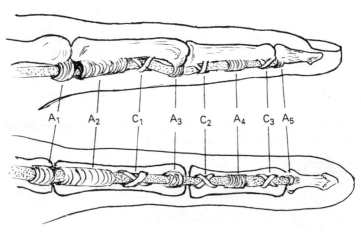

Figure 2.1 *Finger flexor tendon pulley system showing the annular and cruciate ligaments*

Just as muscles need contractility, so tendons must glide, and they do so through synovial sheaths containing synovial fluid. These sheaths lie in the fibro-osseous tunnels (Figure 2.2).

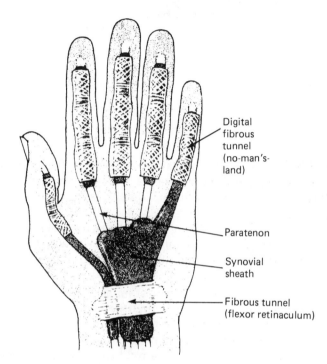

Digital
fibrous
tunnel
(no-man's-
land)

Paratenon

Synovial
sheath

Fibrous tunnel
(flexor retinaculum)

Figure 2.2 *Flexor tendon sheaths*

Nutrition

Tendons receive nutrition from the synovial fluid and the blood supply. The blood supply to a flexor tendon is derived from three sources:

1 Proximal palmar vessels at the muscle-tendon junction.
2 Vincula longa and vincula brevia.
3 Distal bony tendinous insertion.

Each tendon has a longitudinally running chief artery (Figure 2.3).

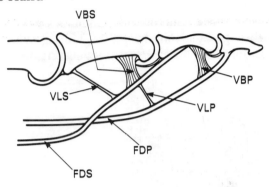

Figure 2.3 *Blood supply of the flexor tendons in the digits: VBS, vinculum brevum to FDS; VLS, vinculum longum to FDS; VBP, vinculum brevum to FDP; VLP, vinculum longum to FDP*

Tendon healing

When a tendon is divided, its ends retract and the wound is filled with haematoma. This haematoma becomes invaded by fibroblasts, from both surrounding injured tissue and the tendon ends themselves. The tendon attempts to heal itself and forms a pseudotendon of fibrous tissue.

Probably, both the tendon ends and the surrounding peritendinous tissues supply fibroblasts which become the new tendon cells. This new fibrous tissue and the inevitable oedema of injury or surgery cause the injured or repaired tendon to adhere within the rigid fibro-osseous tunnel, especially in the digit, or to the palmar fascia.

Tendon repair

The divided tendon ends are repaired as accurately as possible, without tension and with the least interruption to the blood supply (Figure 2.4). Peritendinous adhesions are minimized by sealing the epitenon with fine 6/0–8/0 sutures. When possible the fibro-osseous tunnel is preserved, but if the repaired tendon does not glide through the tunnel, some of the ligament system is excised.

A tendon graft may be either a bridge graft, i.e. between two tendon ends, or a complete replacement attached to muscle

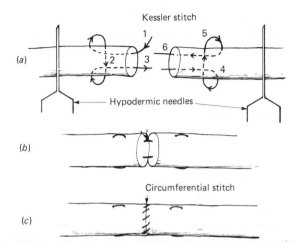

Kessler stitch

Hypodermic needles

Circumferential stitch

Figure 2.4 *Technique of flexor tendon repair. Note the Kessler stitch (4–0 Ti-Cron) grasping the tendon ends; this is less likely to strangle the blood supply than crisscross or zigzag sutures. A circumferential fine 6–0 Prolene suture seals the repair and prevents loose tendon ends adhering to the surrounding structures*

proximally and the phalanx distally. It is sutured either directly to the bone or to a tendon stump.

All key pulleys are preserved or reconstructed to maintain efficient tendon function.

Timing of tendon repairs

The timing of repairs is categorized in the following way:

1 Primary repair: within 12–24 h of injury; suitable for clean, sharp injuries.
2 Delayed primary: 24 h–10 days.
3 Early secondary: 10 days–4 weeks.
4 Late secondary: after 4 weeks.

Delayed primary and secondary repairs are indicated in the case of a dirty or contaminated wound. Late secondary repairs have a tendency to do poorly because of the complications of scarring, the swelling of tendon ends and shortening of the muscle-tendon unit.

Where tendon damage is associated with damage to other tissues, e.g. skin, bones or neurovascular structures, the tendons are best managed by reconstruction at a later date involving two-stage tendon grafting.

Postoperative management

Flexor tendons are most commonly lacerated (or rupture) in zones 1, 2, 3 and 5 (Figure 2.5).

Discussion of the postoperative management of zone 5 is covered in Chapter 4 under 'Postoperative care of nerve repair with tendon involvement'.

Surgery and aftercare of tendon injury in zones 1 and 2 ('no-man's-land') have always been fraught with difficulties, owing to the fact that the tendons lie within the confines of the annular ligaments and the digital sheath. They are therefore prone to adhesion formation.

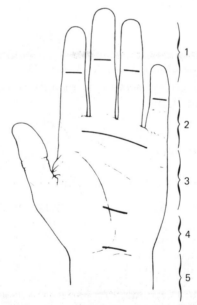

Figure 2.5 *The five zones of flexor tendon injuries. 1, distal to the superficialis insertion; 2, so-called 'no-man's land' in the area of the fibrous flexor sheaths where both tendons are present in a tight tunnel; 3, lumbrical origin; 4, carpal tunnel; 5, proximal to carpal tunnel*

The postoperative management of tendon repair in zones 1 and 2 varies considerably from unit to unit. Management ranges from the conservative, where the hand remains totally immobilized for the first 3–4 weeks, to the radical, where active movement of the repaired tendon commences within days of surgery.

The method employed by the authors is based on Kleinert's controlled active mobilization technique. This method uses rubber band traction with the rubber band being attached to the finger nail (Figure 2.6a). The rubber band flexes the digit passively

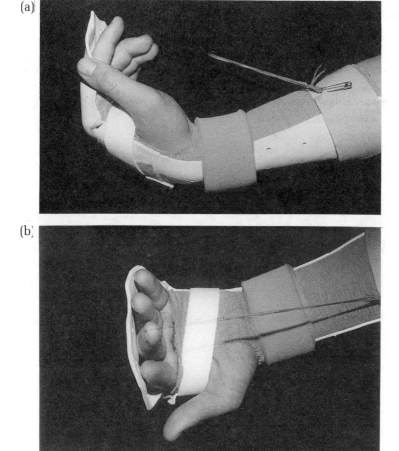

(a)

(b)

Figure 2.6 *(a) Use of rubber band traction following flexor tendon repair in zone 2. (b) Patient is encouraged to extend the IP joints actively against the gentle resistance of the rubber band*

and the patient is permitted actively to extend the IP joints against the gentle resistance of the band (Figure 2.6b).

This system allows a controlled degree of tendon excursion without stressing the repair, with the aim of minimizing adhesion formation.

Ultimately, specific instruction rests with the attending surgeon and will depend on such factors as the site of the repair (especially in relation to pulleys), the quality of the blood supply and the age of the patient.

Aims of therapy

1 To prevent joint stiffness by:
   (a) Initiating early passive flexion of the IP joints.
   (b) Practising early active IP joint extension against the rubber band traction to prevent PIP joint contracture.
2 To regain maximum active flexion range and ensure good return of function.

Days 1–3

The dressing is removed and the wound checked for oedema and

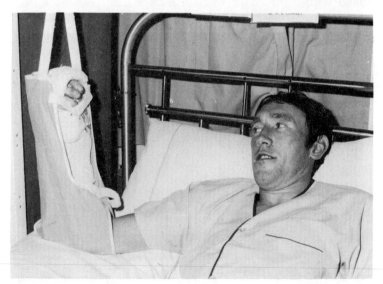

Figure 2.7 *Elevation of the hand in a bedside sling following flexor tendon surgery*

undue tightness of the sutures. The surgeon informs the therapist of the type of repair, its probable strength and its position within the tendon mechanism.

If oedema is present, ice therapy is commenced. The hand is elevated in a sling while the patient is in bed and in a high triangular sling when the patient is ambulant (Figure 2.7).

Splintage

On the third postoperative day the plaster cast is replaced by a lightweight thermoplastic splint maintaining the hand in the following position:

1 Wrist in 35–40 degrees of flexion.
2 MCP joints in 40–50 degrees of flexion.
3 IP joints in neutral extension.

NB If there is any tension on the tendon, nerve or artery repair the MCP joints are positioned in 70 degrees of flexion.

Day 3–week 2

During therapy sessions, passive IP flexion exercises are performed within the limits of pain (Figure 2.8). The IP joints are

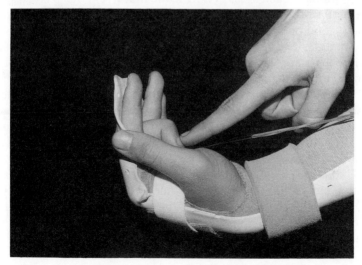

Figure 2.8 *Passive IP joint flexion exercises are practised by the patient inside the splint. This may initially be limited by pain and/or oedema*

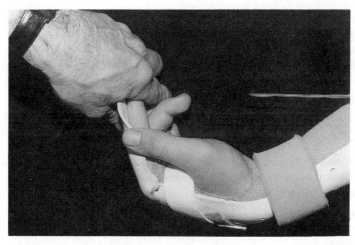

Figure 2.9   *If the FDS is intact it is exercised by holding the MCP joints flexed and trapping the DIP joints of the unaffected digits in extension*

then extended against the resistance of the rubber band, ensuring that the wrist and MCP flexion positions are maintained (Figure 2.6b).

These exercises are carried out on a 2-hourly basis with 5–10 repetitions at each session during the first week; the exercises can be performed on an hourly basis when the wound has settled in the second postoperative week.

Shoulder and elbow movements are carried out several times daily with special attention being given to internal rotation as this is the first movement to be affected in a shoulder problem.

If flexor digitorum superficialis (or sublimis) (FDS) is intact, this muscle is exercised by trapping the distal interphalangeal (DIP) joints of the unaffected fingers in extension and gently flexing the PIP joint of the affected digit (Figure 2.9). This maintains glide of the unaffected tendon.

Under certain circumstances the surgeon may request early active movement of a repaired tendon. This depends on the type of injury, the age of the patient, the security of the repair and its blood supply, and the position of the repair in relation to the annular ligaments (or pulleys).

Any active movement is preceded by full passive flexion warm-up exercises and the movements practised are gentle gross flexion, never stabilized IP flexion movements.

These gentle active flexion exercises are only practised three times per day with only two movements per session, i.e. six flexion movements per day.

It must be stressed that these early active movements are only ever performed at the request of the surgeon.

Weeks 2–3

1 The sutures are removed between days 10 and 14.
2 A warm Lux bath is given before treatment to cleanse the wound, meanwhile ensuring that wrist and MCP joint flexion are maintained.
3 Lanolin massage is commenced to soften scar tissue and increase circulation. The patient is asked to repeat this manoeuvre six times daily for a period of 5–10 min at each of these sessions.
4 Passive IP flexion and active extension exercises are maintained on an hourly basis, with ten movements per exercise session.
5 If digital oedema persists, 2.5 cm Coban wrap is applied very carefully in a distal to proximal direction; it is important to ensure that the digit is not passively extended during this manoeuvre (Figure 2.10).

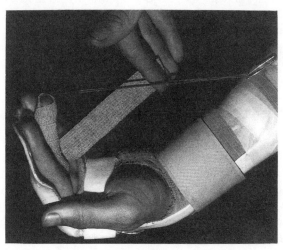

Figure 2.10 *For persistent digital oedema 2.5 cm Coban wrap is carefully applied to the finger, ensuring that it is not passively extended during this manoeuvre*

6 If a PIP flexion contracture appears to be developing in spite of the IP extension exercises, a well-padded dorsal finger splint is applied.

The distal strap of this splint should not encroach on the DIP joint or distal phalanx. In other words, the extension pull (which should be extremely gentle) should be confined to the PIP joint.

As with any splint, the therapist must ensure that there are no pressure points.

Weeks 3–4

1 Gentle active wrist flexion exercises are commenced.
2 Passive flexion exercises are maintained.
3 With the MCP joints stabilized in slight flexion, i.e. approximately 30 degrees, gentle unresisted IP flexion exercises are begun. Five movements every 2 h are recommended at this stage, upgrading the repetitions to ten each hour in the following week (Figure 2.11). These specific finger exercises are

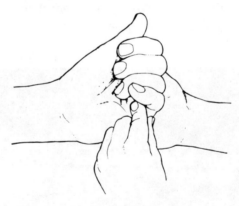

Figure 2.11 *Between the third and fourth postoperative weeks, gentle active IP joint flexion is begun*

followed by gentle gross flexion of all fingers. NB If the repaired tendon is gliding very easily at 3.5 weeks, it is protected for at least another week as scar tissue formation has not been very well established.
4 Active flexion range is now recorded as a baseline.

Weeks 4–6

1 With the wrist held in slight flexion, gentle extension of the digit at all three finger joints is begun.
2 Unresisted active wrist extension is commenced at the beginning of the fifth week, initially with the fingers flexed, and progressing gradually over the next 2 weeks to wrist extension with finger extension.
3 Stabilized IP flexion exercises are maintained.

Weeks 6–8

1 At 6 weeks the protective splint is used only for travelling and sleeping until the end of the eighth week.
2 Active IP flexion range continues to be recorded together with digital extension range.
3 Gentle resistance to active IP flexion is commenced.
4 PIP flexion contractures should ideally have been corrected by this stage. If this is not the case, a dynamic outrigger can be fitted at week eight (Figure 2.12).

   The tension of the elastic band should be minimal at this stage; a tension of 50–100 g would be safe and can be gauged with a spring scale.

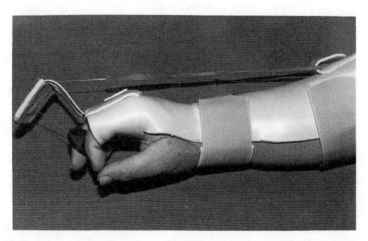

Figure 2.12 *Dorsal dynamic outrigger is used to overcome a PIP joint flexion contracture; this measure is not employed until the eighth week and elastic band tension should be minimal, i.e. a tension of no more than 50–100 g*

5 Lightly resisted functional activity is begun; everyday utensils can be slightly built up as a temporary measure where active flexion range is insufficient to achieve a proper grip.

For those patients involved in specific trades, the therapist can simulate work tasks in the therapy setting as well as giving the patient a home programme.

A leather double fingerstall is useful in achieving grip control if a digit has normal passive flexion range but some limitation of active flexion range (Figure 2.13).

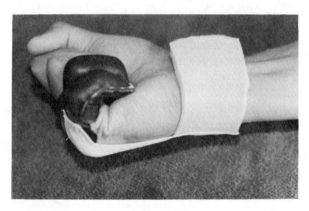

Figure 2.13   *When using the hand in normal gripping activities, a leather double fingerstall is used if there is some limitation in the active flexion range*

Weeks 8–12

1 The splint is discarded, except in the case of schoolchildren who are protected at school until the tenth week.
2 Resisted exercises and activities are upgraded gradually until at 12 weeks maximum stress can be applied.
3 Pinch and power grip strengths are recorded in the last few weeks of treatment to assess progress.

While substantial gains in active flexion range are achieved in the first 3 months after operation, further gains are anticipated during the next 12–18 months and patients should be encouraged to persevere with stablized resisted flexion exercises and resisted activity following discharge from formal therapy.

Flexor pollicis longus repair

Splintage

1 Wrist in slight flexion, i.e. 20–30 degrees.
2 MCP joints in 30 degrees flexion or with the thumb tip in line with the middle finger.
3 The splint should extend to the tip of the thumb and allow extension of the IP joint.

An attempt is made to maintain the thumb in palmar abduction to minimize thumb web tightness. The splint is removed in the direction of the palm, to prevent passive extension of the thumb.

Day 3–week 2

1 If the wound is stable, passive IP flexion is begun with the MCP joint held in full flexion.
2 Gentle active resisted IP extension is practised with the MCP joint held in full flexion.
3 With the thumb held in line with the middle finger, gentle active assisted abduction and adduction are practised to minimize thumb web contracture.

Weeks 2–3

1 As with finger flexor tendon repairs, the tendency to flexion contracture should be checked and a dorsal thumb splint applied if indicated. Tension on the straps is minimal.
2 By the end of the third week gentle active stabilized IP movements are commenced. (Many patients experience difficulty in regaining active IP flexion. Instead of using the extrinsic flexor pollicis longus (FPL), the intrinsic (thenar) muscles are used. This tendency should be controlled because it becomes a habit that is difficult to reverse.) The remainder of the therapy and activity programme follows as for flexor digitorum profundus (FDP) repair.

Week 5 onwards

A C-splint can be used gradually to stretch a tight thumb web at 5 weeks. It is worn first in abduction (Figure 2.14) and then in extension by week 6 or 7.

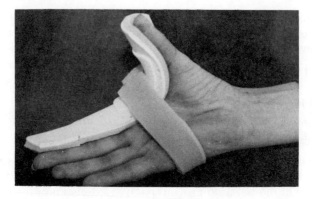

Figure 2.14   *Serial C-splints are used to treat thumb web contracture*

Two-stage tendon reconstruction

Owing to the long-term therapy involved in two-stage tendon reconstruction, patient selection is vital in terms of:

1 Ability to understand the aftercare regimen.
2 Economic and personal commitment to a long-term programme.

Preoperative requirements

1 Full passive flexion.
2 Full digital extension.
3 If the FDS is intact, maximum active PIP movement.

Assessment is performed by all members of the team, namely the surgeon, physiotherapist and occupational therapist.

Technique

When the fibro-osseous tunnel of a digit is so damaged that a repaired or grafted tendon is unlikely to glide satisfactorily along it, the tendon mechanism is excised.

A Silastic rod is attached to the distal tendon stump distal to the DIP joint, and threaded along the digit and through the carpal tunnel to lie freely and proximal to the wrist.

Annular ligament pulleys are reconstructed over the rod, a

fibrous pseudosheath forms around the rod, and after 8–10 weeks the rod is removed and a tendon graft threaded along the tunnel. At the time of insertion of the rod, the muscle motor is anchored to the adjacent muscle-tendon unit if the FDP is involved or to the flexor retinaculum if the FPL is involved, in order to maintain its tone.

Other operative aims may include:

1 Restoration of skin cover, e.g. scar correction.
2 Nerve repair or graft.
3 Capsulotomy to improve the range of motion at the joint.
4 FDS repair or tenolysis.

Precautions

1 The patient must guard against injury. The rod is a large foreign body and is liable to infection and dislodgement.
2 The hand is rested in a volar splint with the wrist in 20–30 degrees extension; the fingers and thumb remain free until the sutures are removed.
3 Heavy resisted use of the hand is avoided while the rod is in place.

Stage 1: postoperative management

Aims

1 To gain full passive flexion and full active extension in the affected digit or digits.
2 To soften scar tissue.
3 To maintain hand function.
4 To maintain full elbow and shoulder movements.

Days 3–14

1 The hand is rested on a volar pan splint with the wrist in slight extension or neutral and the fingers in almost neutral extension. No passive IP joint flexion exercises are performed during the first 2 weeks after surgery; this immobility of the digit is to safeguard against an inflammatory response.
2 Oedema is managed by way of elevation and cold therapy.
3 The mobility of adjacent finger joints is maintained during this

period, ensuring that the digit housing the rod is not aggravated. The wrist is rested during this time.

Day 14

1 The sutures are removed and lanolin massage to the scar is commenced.
2 Gentle active wrist flexion and extension exercises are commenced.
3 Passive IP flexion exercises within comfortable limits are begun.
4 Active finger extension exercises are carried out.
5 The patient is taught how to trap the affected digit with an adjacent one when exercising and during light activity.
   A Velcro buddy strap (Figure 2.15) prevents injury, maintains flexibility and enhances hand function.

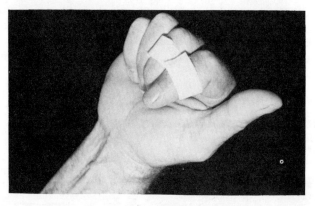

Figure 2.15 *Velcro buddy strap holds the affected finger against a normal digit, thereby maintaining flexibility and preventing injury*

6 Digital oedema is treated with a Lycra pressure fingerstall (Figure 2.16) or 2.5 cm Coban wrap.
7 If the rod has been inserted into the thumb, there is a risk of thumb web contracture. A C-splint is used to overcome any tightness.
8 A flexion strap (Figure 2.17) is applied if there is IP joint stiffness that cannot readily be overcome with passive flexion exercises.
9 The full length of the scar is massaged before each treatment

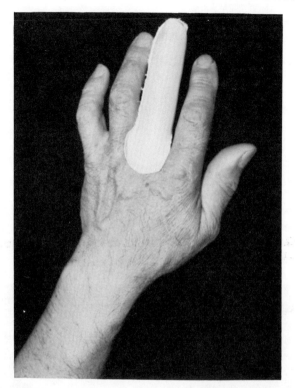

Figure 2.16 *Digital oedema is controlled with a Lycra fingerstall which is applied when the wound is healed*

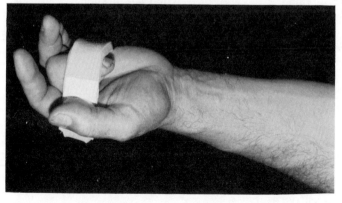

Figure 2.17 *IP joint stiffness is treated with a flexion strap as an adjunct to exercise*

and the patient is instructed to carry out massage six times a day for 10 min each session.

Soft tissue mobility, full active extension and virtually full passive IP joint flexion must be gained before the second stage of surgery.

Full passive flexion may not be possible owing to the bulk of the Silastic rod.

Stage 2: postoperative management

The aftercare regimen is as for primary direct repair. However, the timing of the various stages is often delayed as there is increased risk of rupture with a grafted tendon due to its more precarious blood supply.

Tenolysis

Any injury or operation that interferes with the smooth gliding surface of a tendon system (flexor, extensor or intrinsic) predisposes that tendon to adhesion to adjacent tissues such as skin, retinacular ligament and bone.

In a tenolysis procedure a tendon is freed from its adhesions to restore its glide. Secondary joint changes (capsule or ligament fibrosis) may also need correction.

Tenolysis is indicated only when comprehensive therapy used for at least 6 months after the tendon injury or operation has failed to restore a useful range of movement. As in two-stage tendon reconstruction, patient selection is vital.

Technique

Tenolysis is often performed under a selective peripheral nerve block, with the patient awake and able to co-operate. In this way the surgeon is able to carry out just enough dissection and freeing to give the desired range of movement.

Preoperative aims

1 To soften the scar.

2 To gain the full passive range of movement.
3 To gain a strong muscle-tendon unit.

Postoperative management

The exercise regimen should be sufficient to promote maximum tendon glide without aggravating oedema. The regimen varies from patient to patient and must be judged accordingly.

Complications

1 Oedema from the injury or surgery.
2 Joint stiffness from oedema and pain.
3 Tendon rupture from an impaired blood supply and diminished tendon nutrition (especially following extensive tenolysis or tenolysis within the fibro-osseous tunnel).

The first 14 days following tenolysis are the most critical in determining a successful result.

Splintage

1 Wrist in comfortable extension.
2 MCP joints in gentle flexion
3 IP joints in extension.

Days 1–3

1 Oedema is reduced by rest, elevation and 2-hourly cold packs whose maximum effect is provided in the first 30 min depending on the room temperature.
2 When the wound condition allows, gentle passive flexion is begun. This is followed by several active stabilized flexion movements. These exercises are carried out twice daily and analgesia is used to minimize discomfort.

Days 3–7

The frequency of exercises is upgraded to six times daily.

Days 7–14

1 The above regimen is continued and the number of active

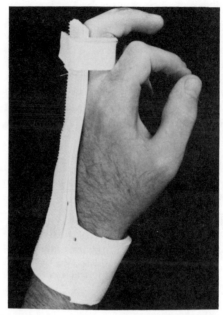

Figure 2.18   *To promote effective flexor tendon glide, an MCP joint blocking splint is worn during active flexion exercises*

flexion exercises is increased to 10–15 movements 2-hourly, providing there is no tissue reaction. (If there is significant tissue reaction, the exercise programme is stepped down. The hand should be rested if crepitus and pain occur as these may be precursors to tendon rupture.)

2 Unresolved oedema is treated with a Lycra pressure fingerstall as soon as the wound is healed.

3 An MCP blocking splint (Figure 2.18) assists in establishing effective flexor tendon glide.

4 The exercise programme is maintained for 3 months, incorporating the treatment methods already described where necessary, i.e. ultrasound, lanolin massage and correction of joint contracture with an outrigger or dorsal finger extension splint.

References and further reading.

Doyle, J. R. and Blythe, W. (1975) The finger flexor tendon sheath and pulleys: anatomy and reconstruction. In *American Association of*

Orthopaedic Surgeons Symposium on Tendon Surgery in the Hand,
C. V. Mosby, St Louis, p. 105

Duran, R. and Houser, R. G. (1975) Controlled passive motion following flexor tendon repair in zones 2 and 3. In *American Association of Orthopaedic Surgeons Symposium on Tendon Surgery in the Hand,* C. V. Mosby, St. Louis

Green, D. P. (ed) (1988) Tendons. In *Operative Hand Surgery,* Vol. 3, 2nd edn, Churchill Livingstone, New York

Hunter, J. M., Schneider, L. H., Mackin, E. J. *et al.* (eds) (1990) Tendons. In *Rehabilitation of the Hand: Surgery and Therapy,* 3rd edn, C. V. Mosby, St. Louis

Kleinert, H. E., Kutz, J. E. and Cohen, M. D. (1975) Primary repair of zone 2 flexor tendon lacerations. In *American Association of Orthopaedic Surgeons Symposium on Tendon Surgery in the Hand,* C. V. Mosby, St. Louis, pp. 91–104

Schneider, L. H. (1985) Flexor tendon injuries. *Monographs on Hand Surgery.* Little, Brown, Boston

Verdan, C. E. (1972) Half a century of flexor tendon surgery. *Journal of Bone and Joint Surgery,* **54A**, 472

3

Extensor tendons

Introduction

Extensor tendons are 'paratenon' tendons and lie in loose areolar tissue on the dorsum of the hand (Figure 3.1). They are thin and

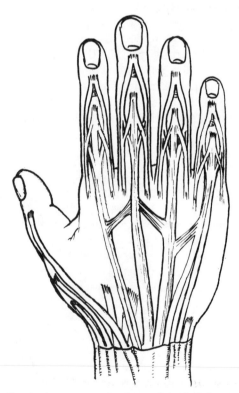

Figure 3.1 *Extrinsic extensor tendons of the hand*

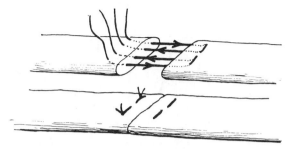

Figure 3.2 *Technique of extensor tendon repair. Mattress sutures are used to prevent the suture material pulling through the longitudinal fibres of the tendon*

flat. When divided, they are repaired with horizontal mattress sutures (Figure 3.2).

Two of the most serious complications of tendon surgery, namely adhesion and rupture, can be even more serious in extensor tendons than in flexor tendons.

To gain good postoperative results, the position of immobilization in the splint must be accurate. Regular review of splinting position will ensure proper maintenance of this correct position.

A loss of glide in the extensor tendon at the level of the MCP and/or PIP joint may result in significant loss of movement of that digit.

Zones of extensor tendon injury and surgery

The extrinsic tendon system of the hand is divided into seven zones for the finger extensors and five zones for the thumb extensors (Figure 3.3).

This division was set down by the Committee on Tendon Injuries for the International Federation of the Society for Surgery of the Hand.

Zones 1 and 2

Injuries to the extensor tendon over the DIP joint and the distal portion of the middle phalanx can be open or closed and will

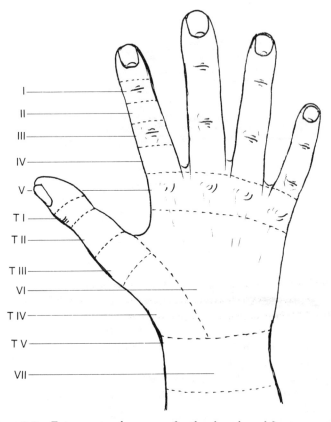

Figure 3.3 *Extensor tendon zones for the thumb and fingers as set down by the Committee on Tendon Injuries for the International Federation of the Society for Surgery of the Hand*

produce the typical mallet deformity, that is a flexion deformity at the DIP joint.

These injuries are frequently associated with a small avulsion fracture at the base of the distal phalanx where the tendon inserts (Figure 3.4).

Closed injuries are treated by a dorsal or volar finger extension splint for 6 weeks; this splint maintains full DIP extension (ideally slight hyperextension), while permitting full PIP joint movement (Figure 3.5).

Patients demonstrating hypermobility of the finger joints will frequently require immobilization of the DIP joint for up to 10–12 weeks.

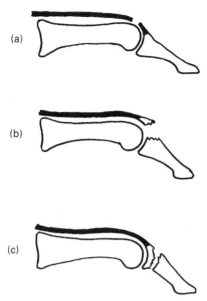

Figure 3.4   *Three types of mallet finger. (a) Rupture of distal extensor tendon. (b) Avulsion fracture of the base of the distal phalanx. (c) Fracture separation of epiphysis of distal phalanx*

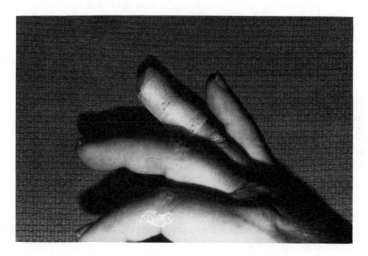

Figure 3.5   *Dorsal or volar DIP extension splint maintains extension of this joint for a minimum of 6 weeks; the splint should permit full PIP joint flexion*

In the case of an avulsion fracture, the splint may need to be placed volarly to avoid painful pressure over the fracture site; also, the splint may need to be changed several times as oedema resolves.

Following the immobilization period, very gentle active DIP joint flexion exercises are commenced, aiming at only minimal flexion during the first week, i.e. 20–30 degrees of flexion. The patient should also attempt gentle DIP joint extension from the flexed position while holding the MCP flexed.

If the flexion deformity appears to be recurring, DIP joint extension splinting is reinstituted for a further 2 weeks when the situation is re-assessed.

Open wounds are best treated by repair and internal fixation of the distal joint with a Kirschner wire which is removed at 2–3 weeks. A dorsal or volar extension splint is then applied until 6 weeks after surgery.

Oedema in the distal segment of the finger can be effectively managed with 2.5 cm Coban wrap.

Good skin condition should be maintained beneath the splint to prevent maceration and the splint should not compromise fingertip circulation.

The patient is shown how to remove the splint at least once a day in order to 'air' the finger. The patient should ensure that the DIP joint is held in full extension during this manoeuvre.

While the splint is off, the skin is gently tapped and massaged to stimulate the circulation.

Zones 3 and 4

Closed or open extensor injuries over the PIP joint produce a buttonhole deformity which, if untreated, becomes a fixed deformity with a PIP joint flexion contracture and a DIP joint hyperextension contracture (Figure 3.6).

This deformity results from the lateral bands falling below the axis of the PIP joint; when this happens the bands become flexors of this joint while at the same time concentrating their extension forces at the DIP joint.

Inability to flex the distal joint is often the most disabling aspect of this deformity.

Suspected closed injuries of the central slip are treated by

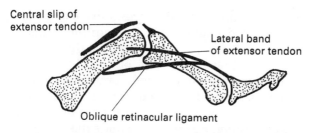

Central slip of
extensor tendon

Lateral band
of extensor tendon

Oblique retinacular ligament

Figure 3.6 *Buttonhole deformity following injury to the central slip of the extensor tendon*

maintaining full extension of the PIP joint for a period of 6 weeks. The DIP joint is left free to move.

PIP joint extension can be maintained by way of (1) a dorsal finger splint, (2) a Capener splint, and (3) plaster cylinder casts. The plaster casts can be changed weekly to monitor skin integrity. Where there is joint oedema, the cast may require second-daily changing during the first week until oedema has stabilized (Figure 3.7).

Before the application of a cast, a film of lanolin is smoothed over the skin for protection.

If the PIP joint cannot be extended passively to neutral extension with ease (i.e. a flexion deformity is present), serial plaster-

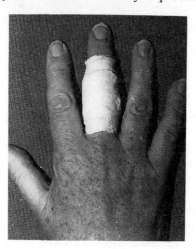

Figure 3.7 *PIP joint can be plaster-casted to maintain full extension. In the presence of a flexion contracture, serial plaster-casting can be carried out until full extension has been regained*

casting is carried out until neutral PIP joint extension has been achieved. Six weeks of PIP joint extension splinting is instituted from this time.

Gentle dynamic traction into flexion of the DIP joint can be incorporated into the plaster cast to help overcome tightness of the oblique retinacular ligament (Figure 3.8).

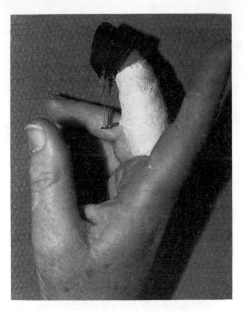

Figure 3.8   *Dynamic traction can be incorporated into the plaster cast to help overcome tightness of the oblique retinacular ligament*

Gentle unresisted active PIP joint flexion/extension exercises are begun following the 6-week immobilization period. These are practised 1–2 hourly with 5–10 repetitions per session.

Open injuries of the central slip are surgically repaired and also require 6 weeks of PIP joint extension splintage.

For the first 3 weeks after operation the PIP joint is held in extension by a Kirschner wire.

For the first few days after operation, the hand is rested in a POSI splint. When oedema and immediate postoperative inflammation have subsided, a well-padded dorsal finger extension splint is fitted for the rest of the immobilization period (Figure 3.9).

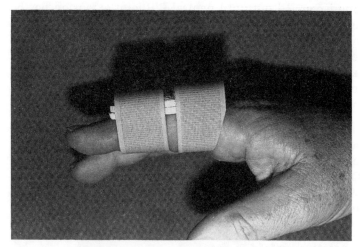

Figure 3.9 *Well-padded dorsal finger splint to maintain extension of the PIP joint*

Early DIP joint flexion exercises are practised to maintain the mobility and length of the oblique retinacular ligament and to promote glide of the lateral bands of the extensor tendon.

Sutures are removed after 10–14 days and scar management by way of lanolin massage is carried out with the joint being held in full extension.

Gentle unresisted PIP joint flexion and extension exercises are commenced at 6 weeks.

Night wearing of the extension splint may continue for several weeks if there is a tendency for the PIP joint to fall into flexion.

Zones 5 and 6

These zones lie between the MCP joints and the extensor retinaculum.

Closed injuries of the sagittal hood system can occur following blunt trauma and lead to an extensor lag or ulnar drift of the tendon.

These injuries are treated by splinting the MCP joints in the extended position for 4–6 weeks.

Common complications

Extensor tendon repairs are often regarded as minor injuries, but there is a significant incidence of:

1 Tendon adhesion.
2 Tendon lag (owing to attenuation of the tendon).
3 Tendon rupture.

Extensor tendon repairs must be treated with as much care and respect as flexor tendons.

The ability of the patient to extend his fingers sufficiently to grasp large objects and also to release them is important from a functional point of view: tendon adhesion and lag can persist for many months.

Postoperative goals include:

1 Good wound care.
2 Oedema control to minimize adhesion formation.
3 Strict maintenance of the correct immobilization position after operation. If splintage is inadequate, some gapping of the tendon ends may occur with resultant lag or failed extension of the MCP joint.

Splintage

The splint is a volar thermoplastic splint which replaces the plaster cast at approximately the third postoperative day and extends from just proximal to the PIP joints to two-thirds along the forearm.

At its distal end, the splint is 'stepped-down' according to the level of each PIP joint to allow for passive exercising of these joints. The position of the splint is as follows:

1 Wrist in 40–45 degrees of extension.
2 MCP joints 0–25 degrees of flexion depending on the surgeon's preference (Figure 3.10).

Days 1–3

The dressing is removed and the state of the wound is assessed. Position within the plaster cast is checked and a thermoplastic splint is fitted as soon as oedema is under control.

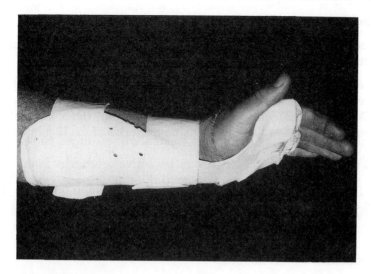

Figure 3.10 *Postoperative splint following repair of the extensor tendon(s) in zones 5 and 6*

The hand should be maintained in high elevation and ice packs used where appropriate.

Instruction is given in the maintenance of shoulder and elbow movements.

Day 3–week 2

With the hand remaining in the splint, gentle passive flexion and extension exercises of the PIP and DIP joints are carried out. Five to ten repetitions every 2 h are usually sufficient to maintain interphalangeal joint mobility.

Weeks 2–4

The sutures are removed and, if the wound is completely healed, lanolin massage is commenced. If scarring is significant, ultra-sound is also commenced; this is carried out using gel and with the hand remaining in the splint.

If the hand has a build up of eschar and devitalized skin, a Lux (pure soap flakes) bath is given; it is important that wrist and finger extension is maintained throughout this procedure.

Weeks 4–6

The hand can be removed from the splint for exercise sessions every 2 h. These exercises include:

1 Gentle active flexion/extension exercises of the MCP joints while IP joint extension is maintained.
2 With the MCP joints maintained in neutral extension, gentle unresisted active flexion/extension exercises of the IP joints are commenced.
3 From week 4–5, the wrist can be actively brought from the extended position into the neutral or 0 degrees extension position; gentle active wrist flexion is begun at the fifth week (the fingers should be in a relaxed, extended position when practising wrist flexion exercises).

Weeks 6–8

The following exercises are added to the programme:

1 Attempting simultaneous flexion of the MCP, PIP and DIP joints, i.e. aiming at making a fist.
2 Extrinsic extension exercises, i.e. practising MCP joint extension with the IP joints held flexed (Figure 3.11).
3 Gentle resistance to extrinsic extension is given at the beginning of the eighth week.

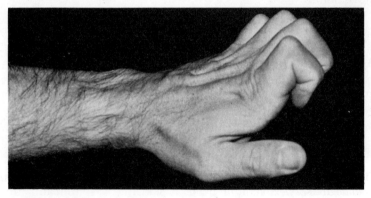

Figure 3.11   *Extrinsic extension exercises*

Weeks 8–12

In this zone of repair, particularly where there is multiple tendon involvement or the injury has been an untidy one with or without a crushing mechanism, it is not uncommon for patients to experience the following difficulties:

1 MCP joint stiffness as a result of immobilization, tendon adherence or dorsal fibrosis.
2 An inability to flex all three finger joints simultaneously, owing to scarring of the dorsal skin.

Stiffness of the MCP joints can be managed by an MCP flexion splint which is not fitted before this time.

Tension of the rubber bands should be gentle, i.e. 100–150 g to begin with.

While the MCP joints are maintained in some degree of flexion by the splint, the patient can practise gentle IP joint flexion exercises.

A flexion strap can be used to overcome final degrees of stiffness at the tenth week, by which time the MCP flexion splint should have achieved a reasonable MCP joint flexion range (Figure 3.12).

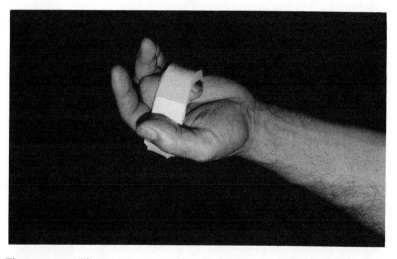

Figure 3.12 *Flexion strap may be used after the tenth week to regain final degrees of flexion*

It may take some time to regain the desired range of movement; the patient should therefore be encouraged to persevere with the exercise and splinting regimen.

Zone 7

This is the area of the extensor tendon beneath the extensor retinaculum.

Here the extensor tendons are prone to proximal retraction. Repaired tendons in this area have a tendency to adhere to one another as well as to the adjacent extensor retinaculum.

Repaired wrist extensors need to be immobilized for at least 4 weeks, and longer if the division is near the insertion of the tendon into the metacarpus.

Postoperative treatment

Splintage

The wrist is splinted in 40–45 degrees extension.

NB If finger extensors have also been repaired, the splint will include the MCP joints as described above.

Day 3–week 2

All finger and thumb exercises are practised to prevent stiffness.

Weeks 2–3

Lanolin massage is commenced when the sutures have been removed and the wound is completely healed.

Weeks 3–5

Active wrist extension exercises are started 3 weeks after the operation.

Active wrist flexion exercises are begun at the fifth week. The splint is discarded between the fifth and seventh weeks and gentle resisted activity is commenced at the eighth week.

Full stress may be placed on the repair after the 12th week.

Repair of extensor pollicis longus

Splintage (Figure 3.13)

1 Wrist in extension.

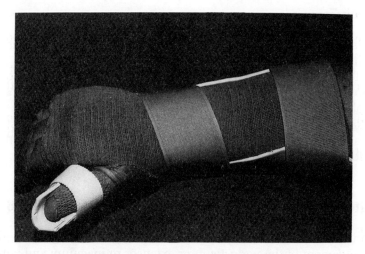

Figure 3.13 *Immobilization splint following repair of extensor pollicis longus*

2 MCP joint extended, not hyperextended (some patients have hypermobility at this joint and a swan-neck deformity of the thumb will ensue if this joint is placed in hyperextension).
3 IP joint extended or hyperextended.
4 The splint extends to just beyond the tip of the thumb.

Day 1–week 4

The hand is rested in the splint; finger joint mobility by way of active flexion and extension exercises is maintained.

Weeks 4–6

The hand is removed from the splint and the thumb allowed to fall into line with the index finger from where it is then actively extended.

Gentle unresisted active flexion and extension exercises of the IP joint are begun. The patient should aim for some degree of hyperextension at this joint if at all possible.

At the beginning of the fifth week, the patient attempts to oppose the thumb to the remaining digits as well as attempting to flex the thumb across the palm.

Week 6 onwards

The thumb is gradually exercised into full flexion and opposition, as well as being actively extended.

The splint is discarded after the sixth week and the patient is warned not to commence heavy lifting until the 12th week after the operation.

If there remains a tendency for the IP joint to fall into flexion, i.e. there is an extension lag, a dorsal extension splint or C-splint worn at night will help control this.

Alternative postoperative regimen for zones 5 and 6

If the extensor tendon injury is considered to be untidy, i.e. with involvement of the periosteum or extensor retinaculum and with adjacent soft tissue injury, a regimen involving gentle glide of the repaired tendon(s) without stress on the repair may be used.

The rationale behind this system is that some 5 mm of tendon excursion without undue tension on the repair helps overcome the tendency to adhesion formation.

This reduces the likelihood of further surgical procedures to free adhesions which often cause limited flexion or extension range.

Following surgery, the hand is positioned in a volar slab with the wrist in extension, the MCP joints in 25 degrees of flexion and the IP joints in full extension.

At 3–7 days after operation when oedema has settled, the volar splint is replaced by a dorsal thermoplastic dynamic outrigger extension splint.

The splint also has a volar component creating a palmar block which prevents the MCP joints from being actively flexed more than 30 degrees.

The wrist is positioned in approximately 45 degrees of extension and the elastic band tension holds the MCP joints at 0 degrees when resting (Figure 3.14).

Days 3–7 to week 4

The patient is taught to flex the MCP joints actively as far as the MCP block, then allow the elastic band traction of the outrigger to extend the fingers passively to their resting position of 0

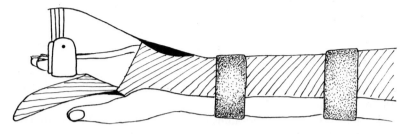

Lateral view

Figure 3.14 *Postoperative dynamic extension splint used in the alternative regimen for an untidy extensor tendon injury in zones 5 and 6*

degrees extension. These exercises are practised ten times every hour.

It may be necessary for the patient to wear dorsal finger extension splints to prevent flexion of the IP joints when carrying out MCP flexion exercises.

Several times a day the IP joints are gently flexed and extended passively; this is done by removing the fingers from the slings and maintaining the MCP joints in neutral extension.

Week 4 onwards

Active MCP joint exercises are now begun and the regimen becomes the same as for 'tidy' tendon repair which has been described.

Alternative regimen for EPL repair

A dynamic outrigger splint is used maintaining the following position:

1 Wrist in 30–40 degrees of extension.
2 Carpometacarpal joint neutral.
3 MCP joint neutral extension.

The elastic traction of the outrigger holds the thumb IP joint at 0 degrees when at rest, while allowing 60 degrees of active IP joint flexion.

The previously described EPL regimen is followed from the fourth week after operation.

References and further reading

Communication: *Second International Meeting of American Society of Hand Therapists*, Boston

Elliot, D. and McGrouther, D. A. (1986) The excursions of the long extensor tendons of the hand. *British Journal of Hand Surgery*, **11**, 77

Elson, R. A. (1986) Rupture of the central slip of the extensor hood of the finger: a test for early diagnosis. *British Journal of Bone and Joint Surgery*, **68**, 229

Evans, R. B. and Burkhalter, W. E. (1983) Early passive motion in complex extensor tendon injury

Evans, R. B. and Burkhalter, W. E. (1986) A study of the dynamic anatomy of extensor tendons and implications for treatment. *American Journal of Hand Surgery*, **11**, 774

Green, D. P. (ed.) (1988) Tendons. In *Operative Hand Surgery*, Vol. 3, 2nd edn, Churchill Livingstone, New York

Harris, C. (1972) The functional anatomy of the extensor mechanism of the finger. *Journal of Bone and Joint Surgery*, **54A**, 7–13

Hunter, J. M., Schneider, L. H., Mackin, E. J. *et al.* (eds) (1990) Tendons. In *Rehabilitation of the Hand : Surgery and Therapy*, 3rd edn, C. V. Mosby, St. Louis

4

Peripheral nerve injuries (including tendon transfers)

Anatomy

Peripheral nerves carry axons from the cell bodies in the central nervous system to the receptor organs in the motor and sensory endplates. Each axon is an extension of the individual cell within the central nervous system (Figure 4.1).

The individual fibres constituting a peripheral nerve are made up of many fine neurofibrils. Most fibres have a fatty coat, or myelin sheath. All fibres are surrounded by a cytoplasmic sheath, the sheath of Schwann, which is a vital covering in the process of degeneration and regeneration.

The endoneurium is the supporting tissue of the individual fibres. The nerve fibres with their related endoneurium form aggregations called bundles, fasciculi or funiculi, which are enclosed by a much larger cellular and collagenous envelope called the perineurium.

The fasciculi are held together by a variable amount of collagenous connective tissue and are enclosed by the outermost envelope, the epineurium.

Each peripheral nerve has a rich intrinsic and extrinsic blood supply. There is a mesoneurium, comparable to a mesotenon.

Types of injury

There are three main types of nerve injury, classified according to

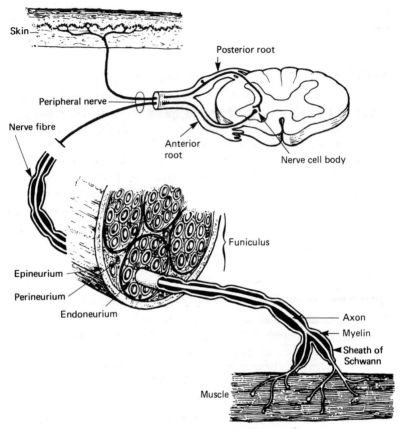

Figure 4.1   *Anatomy of a nerve cell showing the cell body and the nerve fibre or axon with its component parts. (From Grabb, 1970, by permission)*

the extent of damage to the axons and the connective tissue sheath.

Neurapraxia

This is nerve concussion with a transient physiological block. Spontaneous recovery occurs within a few weeks. Anatomical continuity is maintained (Figure 4.2a).

Axonotmesis

This is rupture of the axons while the sheath remains intact.

Spontaneous recovery usually occurs but may take many months (Figure 4.2b).

Neurotmesis

This is partial or complete division of the axons together with the sheath (Figure 4.2c). Recovery is possible only after surgical repair. When there is complete nerve division, the distal segment undergoes wallerian degeneration, i.e. the axons degenerate but the connective tissue sheath remains patent to accept any regenerating fibres that find their way from the proximal end. The proximal end usually forms a neuroma which must be excised before repair.

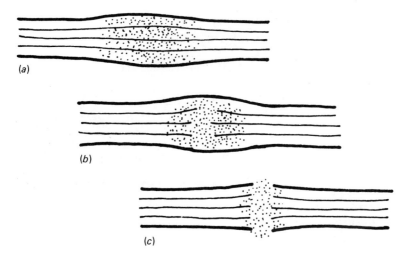

(a)

(b)

(c)

Figure 4.2 *Microscopic types of nerve infury. (a) Neuropraxia: concussion. (b) Axonotmesis: sheath intact, axons severed. (c) Neurotmesis: sheath and axons severed*

Reaction to injury

Following nerve injury, there are changes in the nerve itself and in associated tissues:

1 Skin. Trophic changes cause it to become dry, shiny, and scaly.
2 Muscle.

(a) Imbalance may lead to deformity and consequent joint contracture.

(b) Atrophy may lead to fibrosis.

3 Blood vessels. Circulatory changes result in cold skin.

Wallerian degeneration

Augustus Volney Waller (1816–70) was an English physiologist who described the disintegrative process that occurs in the distal segment of the divided nerve.

After injury, degeneration of the nerve occurs to the level of the proximal node of Ranvier. The distal portion of the axon and the myelin sheath degenerates and the subsequent debris is removed by macrophages (Figure 4.3).

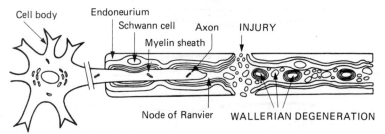

Injury causes degeneration of axon and myelin sheath distal to the wound, and proximally to the next node of Ranvier

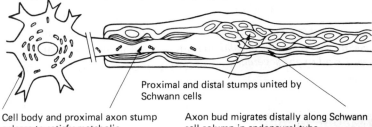

Cell body and proximal axon stump enlarge to satisfy metabolic requirements for regeneration

Axon bud migrates distally along Schwann cell column in endoneural tube

Figure 4.3 *Nerve degeneration and regeneration. When there is complete nerve division, the distal segment undergoes wallerian degeneration, i.e. the axons degenerate but the connective tissue sheaths remain open to accept any regenerating fibres from the proximal nerve end*

Regeneration

Following nerve repair, the proximal and distal stumps are united by Schwann cell proliferation. This proliferation extends down the endoneural tube along which the axon buds migrate.

Nerve repair

The aim of nerve repair is to join as accurately as possible the component connective tissue tubes so that proximal axons regenerate down the distal connective tissue tubes. The more accurate the matching of sensory to sensory and motor to motor nerve fibres, the better is the potential reinnervation of the end organs (Figure 4.4).

Using the operating microscope it is possible to obtain fairly accurate junctions of fascicles, but because of the intertwining and crossing over of nerve fibres it is almost impossible to match fibres with 100% accuracy.

Timing of nerve repair

In recent clean wounds, primary nerve repair is indicated. In untidy wounds, delayed repair is preferable because at 3–6 weeks, when the tissues are healed and pliable, it is easier to ascertain the degree of scarring of the nerve ends to be resected.

Healing

The repaired nerve sheath, whether epineurium or perineurium, takes 3–4 weeks to gain sufficient tensile strength to withstand stress. During this time the repair is splinted.

Nerve grafts

If on approximation of the two nerve ends there is tension, a nerve graft is indicated.

Tension on the repair will impair the blood supply essential to healing.

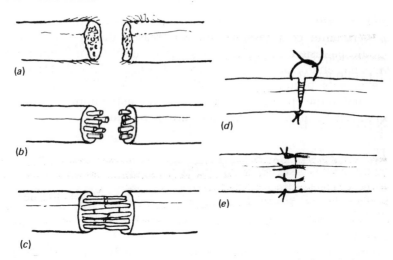

Figure 4.4   *Technique of nerve repair. (a) Cut nerve before dissection. (b) Stripping the perineurium and epineurium and displaying the fascicular bundles. (c) Fascicular repair using 9–0 or 10–0 sutures. (d and e) Epineural repair*

Nerve grafts can be taken from the sural nerve, the dorsal nerve of the foot or the medial cutaneous nerve of the forearm.

It is more difficult to match like axons than in direct repair. However, because there is complete absence of tension, joint mobilization can commence earlier.

Neurolysis

Neurolysis is surgical freeing of a scarred nerve. Common examples include:

1 Median nerve at the carpal tunnel.
2 Ulnar nerve at the cubital tunnel (elbow).
3 Ulnar nerve at Guyon's canal (wrist).

Neurolysis may be performed at various levels. Commonly, as in carpal tunnel syndrome, there is external compression of the epineurium from proliferative flexor tenosynovitis or, in the case of the ulnar nerve at Guyon's canal, by a compressive ganglion. Removal of the external compression is usually sufficient to release the pressure on the congested nerve. (Haematoma, infection or scarring is likely to result in a recurrence of the epineural or perineural compression. For this reason the operative area should be rested in a splint and elevated until the inflammatory response and/or oedema has subsided completely; only then are movements begun.) Occasionally fibrosis is not external but internal to the epineurium, i.e. around the nerve fibres, requiring an internal neurolysis to free the various bundles.

Clinical signs of nerve damage

Motor, sensory and vasomotor changes may be evident after nerve injury.

Motor

Paralysis leading to wasting may be seen in axonotmesis or neurotmesis. Wasting becomes obvious at 4–6 weeks, develops rapidly at 2 months, and reaches its maximum 3 months after nerve injury.

Muscles become fibrotic after about 2 years if reinnervation does not occur.

Sensory

All types of sensation (pain, touch, temperature, stereognosis and two-point discrimination) apart from joint position sense (proprioception) are lost.

Owing to sensory overlap, the area of complete sensory loss contracts soon after injury. Initially, affected skin is dry and scaly.

Vasomotor

Circulatory changes occur in two phases:

1 An early warm phase immediately follows nerve division, as a result of vasoconstrictor paralysis.
2 After 3 weeks the skin becomes cold.

Because of disuse and reduced circulation, atrophy of the skin and nail changes can be observed.

Skin scaliness gradually disappears and the texture of the skin becomes smooth and shiny.

Preoperative care for delayed primary repair or nerve graft

Before surgery is undertaken, it is essential for the hand to be in optimum condition. There should be:

1 Full range of passive movement in all joints. The patient is instructed in exercise techniques so that movements can be practised several times a day.

2 Minimal tendon adherence in the scar area. This can be achieved by a programme of intensive active stabilized movement of individual joints.

3 Good skin condition. Because of the lack of sweating and sebaceous secretion, the skin becomes dry and scaly. It is therefore nourished with lanolin or a rich hand cream several times daily, especially in cold weather or after the hand has been in water.

   The patient is educated to use precautionary measures aimed at avoiding injury from:
   (a) Sharp instruments.
   (b) Heat (e.g. hot water, cooking appliances, cigarettes and radiators).
   (c) Pressure areas and friction burns.

   Should a burn or cut occur then every measure to aid healing is used, as wounds to anaesthetic skin have poor healing ability and a tendency to infection (Figure 4.5). Wounds must be kept clean and dry at all times.

   Until sensory function has returned, the patient is taught to compensate visually.

   Methods of protection include using an insulated mug for hot drinks, well-padded mittens when working in the kitchen, long handled cooking utensils and raised knobs on saucepan lids. In cold weather patients should wear warm gloves or mittens.

4 Correction of deformity or contracture by appropriate splintage. In the presence of an established MCP extension contracture or PIP flexion contracture, an MCP flexion splint or PIP outrigger is indicated. Soft tissue tightness, for example of a flexor muscle-tendon unit, can be gradually stretched using a volar pan splint.

5 Intact musculature should be at optimum strength.

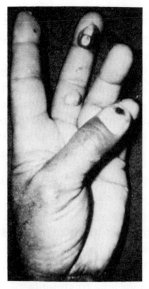

Figure 4.5 *Injury to anaesthetic skin as a result of contact with a hotplate*

Early postoperative care without flexor tendon involvement (weeks 0–4)

After a median or ulnar nerve repair at wrist level, a dorsal splint is used to hold the wrist in sufficient flexion to avoid stress on the repair. The splint should extend just beyond the tips of the fingers with the thumb remaining free.

This splint remains in place for 3–4 weeks, by which time the connective tissue should have sufficient strength to withstand movement of the wrist.

Maintenance of joint mobility and tendon glide

In the absence of flexor tendon repair, the finger and thumb joints of the hand can commence gentle active exercises 2–3 days post-surgery. This prevents joint stiffness and tendon adherence at the site of healing.

Exercises are performed in the splint to ensure maintenance of wrist flexion.

Care of the wound

When the sutures are removed, at about 2 weeks, ultrasound and lanolin massage are commenced.

Initially, massage is carried out very gently. As tolerance to touch and scar condition improve, massage becomes more intensive. The patient is taught how to perform massage and encouraged to carry this out independently six times a day.

Ultrasound and massage reduce the degree and density of scar tissue and assist in desensitizing the neuroma at the site of the repair or graft.

Patient education

This is an important aspect in the management of patients with a peripheral nerve lesion.

Patients should be told:

1 The reasons for the various treatments.
2 That wasting of muscles increases in the early stages following nerve repair.
3 The average rate of nerve regeneration, i.e. about 1 mm per day, and what function may be ultimately expected.
4 That paraesthesia (tingling or pins and needles) and hyperaesthesia (extreme sensitivity) may occur and are normal manifestations of nerve regeneration which will diminish with time and with use of the hand.

Later postoperative care without flexor tendon involvement (week 4 onwards)

1 Care of the anaesthetic skin is continued. If the wound scar is raised and dense, serial silicone elastomer moulds are applied beneath a pressure bandage until scarring is resolved (Figure 4.6).
2 The previous exercise programme is maintained. Gentle active wrist flexion and extension exercises are commenced. Wrist extension is carried out initially with the fingers held flexed, working gradually over the next 2 weeks towards wrist extension with finger extension.

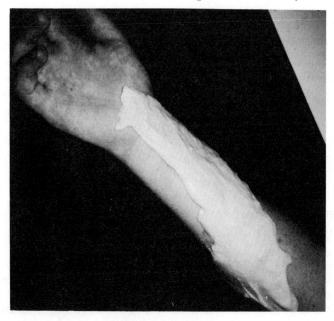

Figure 4.6 *Silicone elastomer mould applied to a raised dense scar*

3 Care of denervated muscle. Muscle length is maintained by passive and active joint movements in the normal planes.

Strength duration curves and electromyography studies assess recovery or regeneration of nerve to muscle. If some sign of recovery is detected, manual muscle testing is also done.

Specific active exercises are given as soon as active muscle contraction is detected.

Hypersensitivity

Sometimes, despite a desensitization programme, hypersensitivity persists at the site of the repair.

If this creates a functional problem when the patient returns to work, a wide forearm cuff (usually 5 cm) that is well-padded (for instance with 7 mm Polycushion) and firmly applied acts as a shock absorber to the sensitive area. The tension of the cuff is controlled by adjusting the Velcro closures.

Early postoperative care with flexor tendon involvement (weeks 0–4)

Splintage

This is as for flexor tendon repair.

Therapy

See Chapter 2 for specific exercises during this time.

Later stage postoperative care with tendon involvement (week 4 onwards)

The major postoperative complication following repair of nerve and tendons is flexor tightness or flexion deformity of the wrist, with or without flexion deformity of the fingers. This is due to the tendons adhering to each other and to surrounding soft tissue. Lanolin massage of the operative scar is performed at least six times daily. This massage is initially gentle to avoid blistering the skin. As tolerance to touch improves over a week or so, massage can become more intensive.

Gentle unresisted flexion exercises of the wrist and finger joints are begun.

To help overcome tendon adherence by promoting effective tendon glide, active finger flexion exercises are stabilized and practised individually. Where possible the wrist is encouraged to assume a more neutral position while the fingers remain flexed.

A cock-up splint is fitted to maintain this less flexed or neutral wrist position. The splint should be worn at night and intermittently during the day.

Over the next 2 weeks the patient practises gentle active wrist extension exercises with the fingers held relaxed, i.e. not attempting to extend the fingers together with the wrist. Conversely, gentle finger extension is practised with the wrist slightly flexed or neutral.

As wrist extension improves, the cock-up splint is modified to maintain gains.

Oedematous hands should be elevated when not being exercised or used. If oedema persists, it should be treated with a Lycra glove.

Week 6

Slight resistance can be applied to flexion exercises and light functional activities are encouraged.

The patient can attempt actively to extend the wrist and fingers together. This may not be possible owing to residual flexor tightness.

If this is the case, the cock-up splint is replaced by a modified POSI splint, with the wrist slightly extended, the MCP joints flexed to comfortable limits and the IP joints extended to comfortable limits. This position provides some stretch to help overcome flexor tightness. The splint need not have a thumb piece (Figure 4.7).

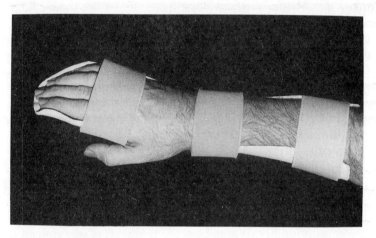

Figure 4.7 *Thermoplastic volar stretch splint is used serially to overcome flexor tightness following repair of nerves and tendons at the wrist*

When this position becomes completely comfortable, the efficacy of the splint as a stretching device has ceased; this may take 1–2 weeks. To provide further stretch, the splint is reheated and flattened out as much as possible to act as a volar stretch splint.

With the wrist in neutral the fingers may still tend to claw. A wide Velcro strap lined with 7 mm Polycushion is applied to exert gentle pressure over the MCP joints while the wrist is maintained in neutral with a wide Velfoam strap.

Over the ensuing weeks the aim is to achieve full digital extension with the wrist in neutral.

When this is possible, the splint can be modified for the last time by placing the wrist in slight extension while at the same time maintaining digital extension. When this is achieved the flexion deformity has been overcome.

Resistance to flexion exercises is gradually increased until at 12 weeks full resistance can be tolerated.

Specific nerve lesions

Median nerve

In a median nerve lesion the hand is referred to as a simian or monkey hand because of the flat appearance of the thenar eminence and the lack of opposition (Figure 4.8).

The thumb lies beside the index finger in the extended and adducted position because of the unopposed action of the extensor pollicis longus (EPL) and the adductor pollicis. In a low (wrist) lesion the following muscles are affected: in the thenar eminence, the abductor pollicis brevis (APB), the flexor pollicis brevis (FPB), and the opponens pollicis (OP); and the first and second lumbricals (MCP flexors).

This results in:

1 Loss of opposition of the thumb.
2 A hyperextension deformity of the MCP joints of the index and middle fingers from overaction of the extensor digitorum communis (EDC).

In a high (elbow or neck) lesion the following muscles are affected in addition: the FPL (anterior interosseous branch of the median nerve), the lateral half of the FDP to the index and middle fingers (anterior interosseous), the pronator quadratus (anterior interosseous), the pronator teres (main branch of the median nerve), the flexor carpi radialis (FCR; main branch), the palmaris longus (PL; main branch), and the FDS (main branch).

The result is:

1 Loss of IP thumb and finger flexion (FPL, all FDS, and FDP to index and middle fingers).
2 Loss of forearm pronation.
3 Weakness of radial deviation of the wrist.

Patients with a median nerve lesion demonstrate clumsiness

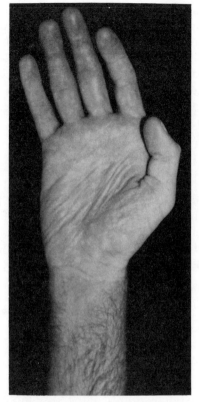

Figure 4.8 *The thumb lies in the adducted and extended position following a median nerve lesion. Note the flattened thenar eminence and trophic changes in the fingertips*

when attempting to pick up either large or small objects. This clumsiness is mainly the result of loss of sensation.

Power grip is affected because of the loss of the stabilizing action of the thumb.

Loss of palmar abduction of the thumb results in the inability to open the hand for grasping large objects, such as a glass.

Trick movement

In a median nerve lesion, pinch grip is obtained by the action of the FPL (in the case of a low lesion) along with the adductor pollicis against the radial side of the index finger.

Lively splint (thumb rotation strap)

The aim of this splint (Figure 4.9) is to bring the thumb into palmar abduction and opposition to facilitate pinch grip.

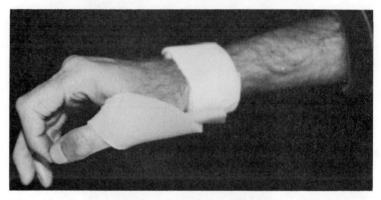

Figure 4.9   *Thumb rotation splint places the thumb in some degree of abduction and opposition, thereby encouraging pinch grip function*

Associated problems

1 Skin injury. This should be taken very seriously (see Care of anaesthetic skin).
2 Reduced thumb web space. This problem can be overcome by a series of well-padded C-splints that gently stretch the web until complete abduction and/or extension have been gained.

Ulnar nerve

An ulnar nerve lesion results in a claw hand whether the lesion is at the neck, elbow or wrist. The MCP joints of the ring and little fingers are held in hyperextension owing to the unopposed action of the EDC and the extensor digiti minimi (EDM) in the absence of the lumbricals (Figure 4.10). (This is known as Duchenne's sign.)

The IP joints are flexed because of overaction of the FDS and FDP, which are unopposed by their antagonists the interossei. In the case of a high lesion, the IP flexion deformity is less marked because of loss of FDP action.

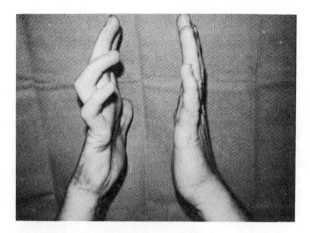

Figure 4.10 *Typical claw deformity in ulnar nerve palsy*

Low (wrist) lesion

The following muscles are affected: in the hypothenar eminence, the abductor digiti minimi (ADM), the flexor digiti minimi (FDM), and the opponens digiti minimi (ODM); the adductor pollicis, all dorsal interossei, all palmar interossei and the medial two lumbricals.

This results in:

1 Loss of finger abduction and adduction, and thumb adduction.
2 Clawing of ring and little fingers as described.
3 Inability to elevate the fifth metacarpal to enable effective opposition between the thumb and little finger.

High (above the elbow) lesion

Together with those above, muscles affected include the flexor carpi ulnaris (FCU) and the FDP to the ring and little fingers. This results in:

1 Weakened ulnar deviation of the wrist because the extensor carpi ulnaris (ECU) is still actively contracting, being supplied by the radial nerve.
2 Loss of flexion of the DIP joints of the little and ring fingers. (Pollock's sign).

In this lesion, power grip is diminished by 50%. This is attributed to:

1 Inability to wrap the fingers fully around an object (because there is no abduction of the fingers).
2 Loss of the elevation of the hypothenar eminence. (Masse's sign).
3 Ineffective clamping action of the thumb in the absence of the adductor pollicis.

Pinch grip is diminished owing to the loss of the first dorsal interosseous muscle and the adductor pollicis. This leads to instability in pinching the thumb against the index finger (Froment's sign).

Trick movements

1 In the absence of the adductor pollicis, adduction of the thumb to the index finger is achieved by the combined action of the FPL and the EPL.
2 In the absence of lumbricals three and four, acute flexion of the IP joints of the ring and little fingers is apparent when attempting to flex the MCP joints of those two fingers.
3 In the absence of the dorsal interossei, abduction of the fingers is mimicked by the EDC, particularly in the index and little fingers which each have an extra extensor: the extensor indicis (EI) and EDM respectively.
4 Adduction of the fingers is mimicked by relaxation of the extensors and contraction of the long flexors.
5 On attempting to oppose the little finger to the thumb, the IP joints of the little finger acutely flex to compensate for a depressed metacarpal owing to the absence of ODM function.

Associated problems

1 Abduction deformity of the little finger. The adductor digiti minimi (ADM) is the first muscle to recover following a lesion at the wrist. As recovery proceeds, the little finger becomes progressively abducted. This posture can interfere with function and is overcome by strapping the little finger to the adjacent ring finger. A Velcro trapper is ideal for this purpose.
2 Hyperaesthesia along the ulnar border of the hand. Hypersensitivity is particularly troublesome to those whose work

involves writing. Patients are encouraged to desensitize the area often during the day by the following physical methods:

(a) Light massage.

(b) Percussion with the fingers of the other hand.

(c) Stimulation with textures, beginning with the least irritating such as cotton wool and gradually progressing to coarser textures like towelling as tolerance improves.

3 Claw deformity. This can be controlled by a 'spaghetti' splint. The principle of this is to support the MCP joints in flexion, thus allowing the long extensors to act on the IP joints in the absence of the intrinsic muscles. (Bouvier's manoeuvre) (Figure 4.11).

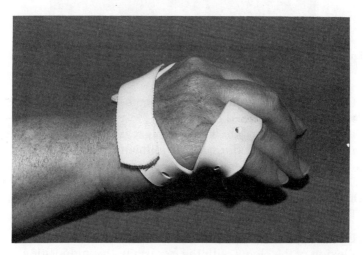

Figure 4.11 *'Spaghetti' splint controls the hyperextension deformity in ulnar nerve palsy, while permitting full flexion and function of the digits*

Radial nerve

The deformity caused by a radial nerve lesion is known as wrist drop (Figure 4.12).

The wrist falls into approximately 45 degrees flexion because the action of the wrist flexors is unopposed by the wrist extensors.

The thumb falls into flexion and palmar abduction because the intrinsic muscles of the thumb are unopposed by the abductor pollicis longus (APL), the EPL, and the extensor pollicis brevis (EPB).

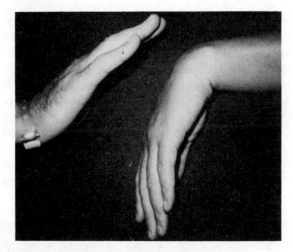

Figure 4.12   *Typical wrist and finger posture in radial nerve palsy*

The MCP joints fall into slight flexion because the action of the lumbricals is unopposed by the EDC.

The most common site of nerve injury is at the radial groove of the humerus. If this is the case, the following muscles are affected: the triceps, the brachioradialis, the extensor carpi radialis longus (ECRL), the extensor carpi radialis brevis (ECRB), the ECU, the EDC, the EPL, the EPB, and the APL.

This results in loss of:

1 Elbow extension (high lesion).
2 Flexion of the elbow with the forearm in the midposition.
3 Wrist extension.
4 Extension of the MCP joints.
5 Thumb extension.

Patients with a radial nerve palsy have a poor grip owing to lack of the stabilizing action of the wrist extensors. They are unable to place large objects on a flat surface because of the loss of wrist extension.

Trick movements

1 There may appear to be contraction of the wrist extensors following strong finger and wrist flexion. This is purely from relaxation of the flexors.

2 Flexion of the MCP joints occurs when the patient attempts to extend the fingers, because the intrinsic muscles extend the IP joints while at the same time flexing the MCP joints.

3 The patient is able to achieve IP thumb extension by palmar abduction of the thumb, owing to the accessory insertion of the abductor pollicis brevis (APB) into the extensor apparatus.

Splintage

A short wrist cock-up splint is worn at all times except during exercise, to prevent straining the wrist joint in the absence of the wrist extensors. (The patient can achieve surprisingly good hand function with the cock-up splint, which places the hand in the functional position. The patient can usually manage sufficient finger extension to release an object by using the intrinsic hand muscles).

A lively splint may also be worn when using the hand. This is a dorsal splint that holds the wrist, fingers and thumb in extension. The tension of the wires or bands is sufficient to maintain thumb and finger extension while allowing active flexion to grasp an object.

Sensory retraining of the hand following median nerve repair at the wrist

Two methods of sensory re-education have been devised: one by C. B. Wynn Parry and the other by A. Lee Dellon and R. M. Curtis. Although methods differ slightly, the aims of retraining in general are the same, i.e. to help patients recognize objects and textures with the altered sensory profile resulting from nerve regeneration.

It is believed that the poor sensory result gained by adults following nerve repair is not so much a failure of surgery but rather that the patient does not achieve his full postoperative sensory potential. Obviously, the age of the patient and the level of motivation are important factors in attaining this potential.

Neurophysiological explanation

The traditional theory of sensory function describes type-specific receptors, namely Krause's end bulbs (temperature), Pacinian corpuscles (pressure) and Meissner's corpuscles (touch). These structures were believed to respond only to specific stimuli.

This theory has been challenged in recent years. It was previously believed that Meissner's corpuscles subserved touch; however, none are to be found in the lips or tongue which are particularly sensitive to touch.

Work on the fate of Meissner's corpuscles following denervation in monkeys (Dellon, 1976) showed convincingly that they could be reinnervated 6–9 months after denervation, but there are no data to show the fate of sensory receptors 2–3 years following nerve division. All the available evidence points to the total disappearance of receptors, and it seems as if the growing nerve terminals create their own receptor system in the periphery.

This evidence has led to the pattern theory, which purports that in handling objects many different receptors are stimulated and that each nerve fibre takes part in many different functions, developing the capacity to transmit information regarding touch, pressure and so on as a result of the demand put on it by active use. Thus the pattern of electrical impulses in the nerve determines the type of sensation rather than any specificity of the end organs.

The particular pattern of discharges arriving at the cord depends on:

1 The number of receptors stimulated.
2 Their frequency response.
3 Whether they are slow or quick in adapting.
4 The sequential nature of their discharges.

Following median nerve suture, there is first, a reduction of fibre density (that is fewer nerve fibres), and secondly, a reduction in the conduction velocity of motor and sensory fibres, which never returns to normal following nerve suture in adults.

These two factors lead to an altered pattern of electrical discharges arriving at the dorsal horn and therefore at the sensory cortex.

Experiments performed by Paul *et al.* (1972) on the Macaque monkey revealed that regeneration following nerve division and primary suture led to marked misrepresentation of the peripheral sensory field in the cortex. Sensory retraining must therefore involve reorganization of central connections.

In response to abnormal stimuli, the patient is taught to lay down new response patterns in the brain. Utilizing preinjury patterns of response stored in the brain the patient relates his abnormal sensation to the nature of the surface of the object tested. Thus the patient is trained to match a new coding of afferent signals (with slower conduction and lower fibre density) with the normal engram previously laid down in the central nervous system.

Sensory retraining technique using the Wynn Parry method

The aim of retraining is to improve stereognostic ability (i.e. the recognition of an object by assessing its shape, weight, size and texture), with the result that functional dexterity improves even though two-point discrimination readings may not show significant improvement.

Sensory retraining is begun as soon as the patient is able to discern moving touch in the fingertips.

The hand is placed behind a screen so that the patient cannot see the test object. To begin testing, a number of differently shaped blocks are placed in the patient's hand. The patient is asked to try to identify the shape by moving the block around in the hand and/ assessing any sharp points or smooth rounded edges. Attempts are also made to judge the weight of the blocks in relation to each other.

If there is failure to recognize the shape, the screen is removed so that the patient can relate what is seen to what is felt, thereby developing a tactile-visual image and in this way retraining the abnormal sensory impulses. When correct recognition of shapes and weights has been achieved, blocks with different textures on one surface are used for testing.

The time taken for correct recognition is noted. In this way, progress can be assessed at regular intervals.

The next stage of retraining involves the recognition of textures (Figure 4.13). To begin with, textures very different from one another are used, such as velvet and coarse sandpaper. As recognition improves, textures with only subtle differences can be introduced.

Even if the patient fails to name the texture accurately, he is encouraged to describe his sensory impressions, e.g. rough, smooth, prickly or spongy. By describing these impressions the patient can often deduce the nature of the texture; he is, in fact,

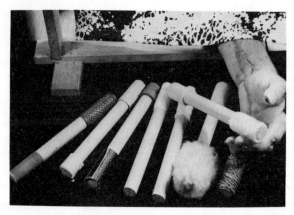

Figure 4.13   *Sensory retraining involving the recognition of textures*

reproducing in slow motion what the normal hand does automatically and quickly. As with the blocks, the time taken for recognition is noted.

The following are examples of textures used for retraining: sheepskin, velvet, corduroy, carpet, pimple rubber, leather, tulle, wool, scouring pad, sponge, sandpaper, silk, towelling, hessian, felt and Laminex. As these are mastered, new textures are included.

The final stage of retraining involves the recognition of everyday objects (Figure 4.14). The objects used for testing should be

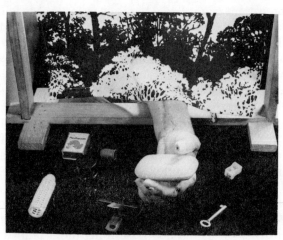

Figure 4.14   *Patient is tested with a variety of everyday objects*

relevant to the patient's experiences, for example a nut or a bolt is generally not a suitable test item for a woman involved in office work.

For initial testing, gross objects are used, such as soap, a matchbox, a tennis ball, an egg cup, a nailbrush, an electric plug and a toothpaste tube.

Because proprioception is a sense that generally remains intact or recovers well, the patient is usually able to gauge the size of an object. By exploring the object slowly, further clues can be gained by assessing shape, texture, temperature and density.

When gross objects have been mastered, finer objects are used, such as a coin, a safety pin, a paper clip, a button, a peg, a matchstick, a nut, a bolt, a hairpin, a hair roller, a marble, a pencil, chalk, a key, a watch and a rubber band.

Training sessions are short (10–15 min) and ideally carried out several times a day.

New textures and objects are added regularly and treatment can be varied by the use of games, e.g. burying objects in sand or sawdust and asking the patient to select specific items.

Localization

Incorrect localization is treated by occluding vision while touching the volar surface of the patient's hand and asking him to identify the point of contact with the index finger of the other hand. If localization is incorrect, the patient is asked to look at the testing point and to relate where he felt the contact to where the stimulus was actually applied.

Following several weeks of retraining, patients usually improve quite dramatically in their recognition times for textures and objects, with an overall improvement in functional dexterity.

The more demands made by the patient on his nerve endings, the faster and more accurate is the response in testing and the greater is the functional dexterity achieved.

Tendon transfers

Where motor recovery has not occurred 18–24 months after nerve repair or where the patient is an adult with a high nerve lesion and motor recovery is deemed unlikely, tendon transfers to regain function are considered. If a tendon transfer is to be successful, there should be adequate sensory recovery.

Definition

A muscle-tendon unit whose function has been lost by injury or disease, e.g. leprosy or peripheral nerve damage, can have its function replaced by transferring an expendable muscle-tendon unit from another part of the limb.

Prerequisites

1 The patient must be a suitable candidate for reconstructive surgery.
2 The muscles to be transferred must be grade 5 voluntary power/strength because first, transferred muscles lose one grade of power as the result of being moved, and secondly, some strength is lost during the initial period of immobilization. If the transfer muscle is weak, a specific resistive exercise programme is instituted. A full muscle chart is drawn up to determine:
   (a) Which muscles have been affected by the nerve lesion.
   (b) Which, if any, of the more proximal muscles have recovered in a high lesion.
   (c) The power of potential transfer muscles.
3 All joints that will be affected either directly or indirectly by the transfer of tendons must be fully passively mobile. Tendon transfers will not move or correct stiff or contracted joints.
4 All skin and soft tissue in the area of the transfer must be pliable and mobile. Any preoperative soft tissue adherence will prevent effective glide of the transferred tendon. Also, any tightness, e.g. thumb web contracture, is corrected before surgery.

Healing of tendon transfers

Tendon transfers are sutured under a degree of tension to maintain a little contractility. To prevent tension on the repair zone the joints must be splinted so as to relax the repair.

The repair is either tendon to tendon or tendon to bone, and requires about 4 weeks of healing before it is safe to subject it to the gentle stress of active movement in the inner range of muscle contraction.

Healing also occurs along the course of the transferred tendon, and adhesions to surrounding tissue (especially around any pulleys) require gentle mobilization by lanolin massage and other therapy measures, such as ultrasound.

Postoperative complications

1 Adhesions along the course of the transfer.
2 Rupture at the junction.
3 Incorrect tension: excessive tension ultimately leads to joint contracture; too much slack or insufficient tension results in ineffective movement.

Postoperative treatment of specific tendon transfers

Ulnar nerve palsy

There are a number of procedures used (both static and dynamic) to correct the 'intrinsic-minus hand' (claw deformity). While the static procedures control the claw deformity, they do not restore power to finger flexion.

Examples of static procedures include:

1 Capsulodesis of the MCP joints: a short flap of the volar plate is sutured into the neck of the metacarpal, holding the MCP joint in 20 degrees of flexion.
2 Flexor pulley advancement. The A2 pulley is split on each side for 1.5–2.5 cm to the middle level of the of the proximal phalanx; this causes 'bowstringing' of the flexor tendon, thus increasing the moment across the MCP joint.
3 Volar tenodesis. A free graft is passed from the central slip insertion at the PIP joint through the lumbrical canal to the deep transverse metacarpal ligament. The tension for each finger is adjusted individually.

Common dynamic procedures

These include:

1 Intrinsic transfer using ECRL which is lengthened with a free tendon graft (palmaris longus or plantaris).

The postoperative management of this procedure (Figure 4.15) is described below.

2 'Lasso' procedure. The FDS of the middle finger is divided into two or four slips and passed volarly through the flexor sheath at the distal edge of the A1 pulley or the proximal edge of the A2 pulley and sutured to itself. One-half of the distal tendon of the donor superficialis is tenodesed across the PIP joint to prevent a hyperextension deformity.

Thumb procedures

To restore thumb adduction and pulp to pulp pinch the following procedures can be performed:

1 Brachioradialis or extensor indicis is transferred to the abductor tubercle of the thumb.
2 Extensor indicis or extensor pollicis brevis is transferred into the tendon of the first dorsal interosseous.
3 Alternatively, a slip of APL is lengthened with either palmaris longus or plantaris and sutured to the tendon of the first dorsal interosseous muscle.
4 An alternative to tendon transfer is fusion of the MCP joint.

Intrinsic transfer using ECRL or ECRB

Preoperative requirements

1 PIP joints must be fully mobile in passive extension and the MCP joints fully mobile in passive flexion.
2 It is important that the patient learns how to extend the wrist while at the same time keeping the fingers completely relaxed, i.e. there should be no finger extension during wrist extension.

Operative procedure

The ECRL is divided at its insertion at the base of the second metacarpal. The graft is lengthened using PL or plantaris and is then divided into two slips. Each slip is passed through its respective intermetacarpal space volar to the deep transverse metacarpal ligament and then attached to the radial aspect of the proximal phalanx of the ring and little fingers. A drill hole is made into which the tendon slip is inserted and held with a pull-out wire (Figure 4.15).

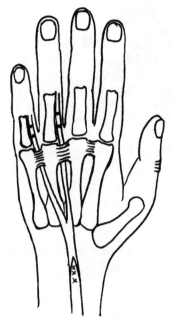

Figure 4.15 *Intrinsic transfer*

Postoperative management

Following intrinsic transfer it is not unusual for patients to experience some degree of pain during the first week after operation. Analgesia at this time is therefore important, particularly before the first change of dressing and splint.

Splintage

The hand is splinted in the following position:

1 Wrist in 45 degrees extension.
2 MCP joints in full flexion.
3 IP joints in full extension.
4 Thumb remaining free (Figure 4.16).

Day 3–week 4

The dressing is removed, the wound is checked and the splint is assessed for comfort and correct position.

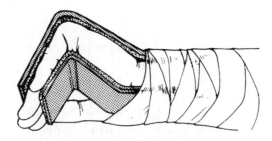

Figure 4.16   *Postoperative immobilization following intrinsic transfer for ulnar nerve palsy*

Week 4

When the hand is removed from the splint there will be a slight relaxation of the positions of wrist extension and MCP joint flexion.

The patient is asked to extend the wrist actively and then to relax. This movement is performed with IP joint extension being maintained. To ensure that the patient achieves this, the therapist places a hand beneath the fingertips during wrist extension.

The action of extending the wrist should produce a measure of MCP joint flexion. This exercise is practised for approximately 1 week or until efficient MCP flexion is gained using the action of ECRL. The exercise should be performed 1–2 hourly with five repetitions each session.

Week 5

The patient now attempts to use the transfers as IP joint extensors. With the wrist extended and maintaining MCP joint flexion, i.e. with ECRL contracted, the patient gently flexes and then extends the fingers.

Once the above exercises have been mastered, they are then practised with the hand in varying positions: namely in pronation, supination, flexion and extension.

Gentle unresisted wrist flexion is also begun at the fifth week.

Weeks 6–12

Light gripping activities may be commenced. If finger flexion is limited, it may be necessary temporarily to build up the handles of everyday utensils such as cutlery.

Graded resistance is applied to MCP joint flexion with the IP joints extended, i.e. intrinsic flexion.

The activity programme is also upgraded to restore maximum pinch and power grip function. The splint is discarded at the eighth week.

Workers involved in heavy manual work may resume normal activities after the 14th week.

Opponensplasty

This is for a low level lesion at the wrist. The tendons most commonly transferred for this procedure include:

1 Flexor digitorum superficialis (FDS) of the ring finger.
2 Extensor indicis (EI).
3 Palmaris longus (PL).
4 Extensor carpi ulnaris (ECU).
5 Hypothenar muscle transfer (using an ulnar innervated intrinsic muscle, abductor digiti minimi).

Preoperative requirements

1 Normal or maximal thumb web span.
2 Mobile thumb joints.
3 Full mobility of the unaffected digits.

Operative procedure using FDS of ring finger

The tendon is sectioned at the level of the PIP joint and is withdrawn just proximal to the carpal tunnel. A pulley is constructed at the distal end of FCU, through which the tendon is passed in a line from the pisiform bone to the MCP joint of the thumb.

The tendon is divided into two slips. One slip is sutured into the insertion of adductor pollicis and the other, more distally, into the extensor apparatus (Figure 4.17).

At the end of the operation, with the wrist extended to 45 degrees, there should be sufficient tension on the transfer for the thumb to lie in complete opposition at the carpometacarpal joint and in complete extension at both the MCP and IP joints.

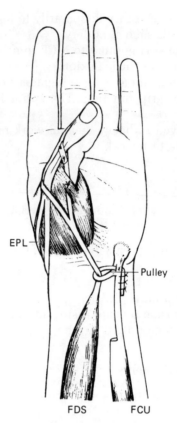

EPL

Pulley

FDS   FCU

Figure 4.17 *Opposition transfer for low median nerve palsy using FDS of the ring finger as the motor*

Postoperative management

Splintage

1 Wrist in neutral or slight flexion.
2 Thumb abducted from the palm and opposed across the palm in line with the middle finger. The splint should extend to the tip of the thumb and hold the IP joint in extension to prevent tension on the suture lines. The fingers are left free to move (Figure 4.18).

Day 3–week 4

On the third day the splint is removed, ensuring at all times that

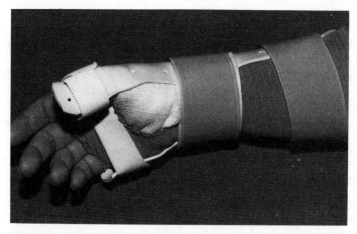

Figure 4.18 *Postoperative immobilization following opposition transfer for low level median nerve palsy*

the thumb is held opposed and that the wrist does not fall into any degree of extension.

The wound is checked and redressed and a thermoplastic splint is constructed.

At 2 weeks the sutures are removed and lanolin massage is begun. This should be performed six times a day by the patient always within the confines of the splint.

Weeks 4–5

Active use of the transferred tendon is begun. The forearm and hand must be well supported and initially the index, middle and little finger DIP joints are trapped in extension as flexion of the ring finger is attempted. This will produce active contraction of the ring finger FDS which pulling on its new insertion will cause a flicker of thumb abduction and opposition.

It may be necessary to repeat this action for two or three treatment sessions until the patient is able actively to contract the muscle and produce spontaneous movement of the thumb.

When this has occurred, the thumb is gently moved actively just past the radial side of the index finger and the patient is asked to abduct and oppose the thumb actively without resistance.

Only when the patient has learnt independent control of the transfer does he practise the exercises on his own.

Weeks 5–7

Active abduction and opposition are practised with the hand in all postures.

Full active thumb extension is gently encouraged and the splint is worn only for travelling and sleeping until the end of the seventh week.

The patient may commence light non-resistive activities to encourage pincer function, e.g. board games, writing and ADL.

Weeks 7–12

Graded resistance is applied to the transferred tendon by way of exercises and graded activity.

The transfer should be able to withstand normal strain at 12–14 weeks after the operation.

Tendon transfers for radial nerve palsy

These are low level, i.e. distal to the elbow. The most common transfers are:

1 Pronator teres (PT) to ECRB
   FCU to EDC
   PL to EPL
2 PT to ECRL and ECRB
   FDS (middle finger) to EDC
   FDS (ring finger) to EI and APL
   FCR to APL and EPB
3 PT to ECRB
   FCR to EDC
   PL to EPL

The postoperative treatment described below refers to the following transfer:

1 PT to ECRB (wrist extension)
2 FCU to EDC (finger extension)
3 PL to EPL (thumb extension)

Preoperative requirements

1 The wrist must be passively mobile in extension.
2 The MCP joints must be passively mobile in extension.

3 The thumb web space must be normal.
4 There must be full range of pronation and supination.
5 There must be full range of elbow flexion and extension.

Operative procedure

1 PT is stripped with its periosteal insertion from the radius, rerouted superficial to the brachioradialis and the ECRL, and sutured to the ECRB as distally as possible.
2 FCU is freed extensively to create a direct line of pull from its origin to its new insertion into the EDC tendons just proximal to the extensor retinaculum (an end-to-side junction).
3 EPL is re-routed out of the extensor retinaculum. The PL is divided at the flexor retinaculum and sutured to the re-routed EPL creating a combined abduction-extension force on the thumb (Figure 4.19).

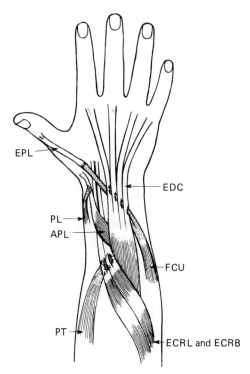

Figure 4.19 *Tendon transfer for radial nerve palsy using pronator teres, FCU and PL as motors*

Postoperative management

Splintage

1 Elbow in 90 degrees flexion.
2 Forearm in pronation.
3 Wrist in full extension.
4 MCP joints in neutral extension. The splint extends as far as the PIP joints, allowing full flexion of the IP joints.
5 Thumb in full extension with the splint extending to the tip (Figure 4.20).

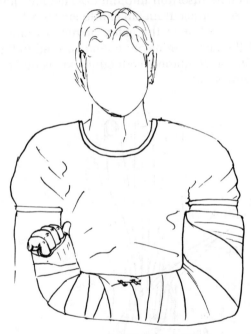

Figure 4.20 *Postoperative immobilization following tendon transfer for low level radial nerve palsy*

Day 3–week 2

The dressing on the dorsum of the hand and forearm is usually removed on the third day and the wound checked. The postoperative plaster is usually replaced with a thermoplastic splint. The splint should be checked for comfort, position and the exclusion of pressure areas.

Because of the extent of surgery, oedema is anticipated and ice therapy is employed until oedema has subsided.

Active flexion exercises of the IP joints of the fingers (not the thumb) are commenced, followed by passive extension of the IP joints.

Weeks 2–4

There is a high incidence of adhesion of the transferred tendons to the dorsum of the forearm and once sutures are removed, it is important that ultrasound and massage are begun.

At home the patient practises active IP joint flexion of the fingers followed by passive IP joint extension.

Week 4

Maintaining elbow flexion, wrist extension, MCP joint extension and thumb extension, the arm is removed from the splint. The patient is asked to:

1 Gently pronate the forearm. This will result in slight wrist extension.
2 Gently flex the wrist. This will result in simultaneous finger and thumb extension.

These exercises are practised under supervision only, until isolated wrist extension without pronation, and MCP joint extrinsic extension without wrist flexion, are achieved. The patient is then able to practise these exercises independently.

Five to ten active movements every 2 h are sufficient at this stage, the hand being rested in the splint in between exercise sessions.

Week 5

During treatment the elbow is gently extended and supination of the forearm is commenced. These movements are performed only under supervision and the arm is returned to the splint directly following treatment.

The MCP joints commence active flexion, initially with the IP joints extended, then working gradually towards gaining full MCP/IP joint flexion simultaneously at 8–10 weeks.

Week 6

The splint is shortened to allow free elbow movement. The above exercises are continued and active wrist flexion exercises are carried out more diligently.

Week 7

The splint is shortened once more to permit MCP joint flexion. The splint is now purely a wrist extension splint, worn when the patient is sleeping or travelling. The hand should be used as much as possible, however, without resistance.

Weeks 8–12

Graded resistance is incorporated into the exercise programme and the splint is discarded at the end of the eighth week.

A normal range of wrist flexion may not be achieved until 6 months after the operation, but the patient is encouraged to practise formal exercise until maximum wrist extension and flexion are gained, and until the adhesions that follow such extensive surgery are reduced to a minimum.

A graded activity programme assists in restoring pinch and power grip function.

Unrestricted activity is allowed after 12–14 weeks.

References and further reading

Beasley, R. W. (1975) Basic considerations for tendon transfer operations in the upper extremity. In *American Association of Orthopaedic Surgeons Symposium on Tendon Surgery in the Hand*, C. V. Mosby, St. Louis, pp. 163–170

Brand, P. W. (1975) Tendon transfers in the forearm. In *Hand Surgery*, 2nd edn (ed. J. E. Flyn) Williams and Wilkins, Baltimore

Conolly, W. B. and Morrin, J. (1981) Sensory rehabilitation of the hand. *Lancet*, i. 135

Curtis, R. M. and Dellon, A. L. (1980) Sensory re-education after peripheral nerve injury. In *Management of Peripheral Nerve Injuries* (eds. G. Omer and M. Spinner), W. B. Saunders, Philadelphia, pp. 769–778

Dellon, A. L. (1976) Reinnervation of denervated Meissner's corpuscles. A sequential histological study in the monkey following fascicular repair. *Journal of Hand Surgery*, i, 98–109

Dellon, A. L., Curtis, R. M. and Edgerton, M. L. (1972) Evaluating recovery of sensation in the hand following nerve injury. *Johns Hopkins Medical Journal*, **130**, 235–243

Dellon, A. L., Curtis, R. M. and Edgerton, M. L. (1974) Re-education of sensation in the hand following nerve injury. *Plastic and Reconstructive Surgery Journal*, **53**, 297–305

Grabb, W. C. (1970) *Orthopaedic Clinics of North America*, **1**, 419

Green, D. P. (ed.) (1988) Nerves and nerve reconstruction. In *Operative Hand Surgery*, vol. 2, 2nd edn, Churchill Livingstone, New York.

Hunter, J. M., Schneider, L. H., Mackin, E. J. *et al.* (eds) (1990) Nerve injuries. In *Rehabilitation of the Hand : Surgery and Therapy*, 3rd edn, C. V. Mosby, St. Louis

Kendall, F. P. (1983) *Muscles – Testing and Function*, Williams and Wilkins, Baltimore

Moran, C. A. and Callahan, A. D. (1986) Sensibility measurement and management. In *Hand Rehabilitation (Clinics in Physical Therapy Series)* (ed. C. A. Moran), Churchill Livingstone, New York, pp. 45–68

Omer, G. E. (1974) The technique and timing of tendon transfers. *Orthopaedic Clinics of North America*, **5**, 243–252

Paul, R. L., Merzescih, M. and Goodman, H. (1972) Representation of slowly and rapidly adapting mechanoreceptors of the hand in Broadmann's areas 3 and 1 of *Macaca mulata*. *Brain Research*, **36**, 229

Seddon, H. J. (1954) *Peripheral Nerve Injuries*, HMSO, London

Smith, R. H. (1987) *Tendon Transfers of the Hand and Forearm*, Monographs in Hand Surgery, Little, Brown, Boston.

Spinner, M. (1972) *Injuries to the Major Branches of Peripheral Nerves of the Forearm*, W. B. Saunders, Philadelphia

Sunderland, S. (1968) *Nerves and Nerve Injuries*, Churchill Livingstone, London

Wynn Parry, C. B. (1981) Peripheral nerve injuries. In *Rehabilitation of the Hand*, Butterworths, London, pp. 78–207

Wynn Parry, C. B. and Salter, M. (1976) Sensory re-education after median nerve lesions. *Hand*, **8**, 250–257

5
Fractures

Classification

1 Closed or open.
2 Stable or unstable.
3 Spiral, transverse or comminuted.
4 According to site, e.g. neck, midshaft or base (Figure 5.1).

Consideration should be given to the force that produced the fracture as this will give an indication of the degree of soft tissue damage.

A direct blow usually results in a transverse fracture, a crushing injury in a comminuted fracture and a twisting injury in a spiral or oblique fracture.

Radiographs should be taken in three views, i.e. anteroposterior, oblique and lateral.

Stability

In a stable fracture the bone fragments do not tend to displace, e.g. incomplete fractures and small marginal joint fractures. Most fractures are stable after reduction. If reduction is necessary then it should be gentle and accurate, take place under adequate anaesthesia, and be followed by radiographs.

Unstable fractures require internal fixation, e.g. fracture dislocations, joint injuries with major ligament rupture and spiral fractures.

Healing process

A fractured bone heals in successive stages (Figure 5.2) as follows:

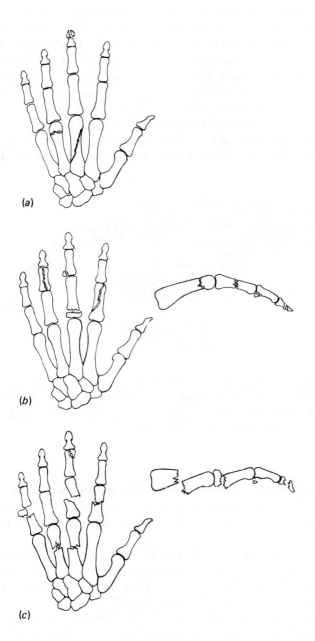

Figure 5.1   *Classification of fractures. (a) Stable. (b) Potentially unstable. (c) Unstable*

1 Procallus (granulation tissue). A blood clot heals the gap between and around the fractured bone ends. The clot coagulates to form the fracture haematoma and this becomes invaded by new vessels and inflammatory cells. The inflammatory cells and the osteoblasts that follow come from the neighbouring tissues, the bone marrow, the periosteum and the muscles. Osteoblasts from the bone proliferate rapidly. The procallus forms in 1–6 weeks depending on the size of the bone fractured and the gap between the bone ends. All neighbouring tissues become inflamed. Radiographs show porosis from hyperaemia.

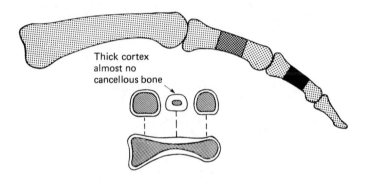

Thick cortex
almost no
cancellous bone

Figure 5.2 *Healing timetable for bone. Fracture consolidation varies within each segment of the hand and is slowest where the ratio of cortical to cancellous bone is highest.* ▦, *3–5 weeks;* ▧, *5–7 weeks;* ■, *10–14 weeks. (From Moberg, 1950, by permission)*

2 Fibrocartilage (osteoid tissue). Within the first week of its formation the procallus begins to differentiate into osteoid tissue which is dense and fibrous. Radiographs still show rarefaction.
3 Bony callus. Within a few days new bone begins to be laid down into the osteoid tissue beginning first as a sheath of subperiosteal and subendosteal bone. About the tenth day after fracture, radiographs show autolysis of the adjacent cortex with resorption and replacement. At about the third or fourth week, bony callus unites across the fracture. This may not show on radiographs until 4–6 weeks.
4 Remodelling with removal of external and internal callus.

Complications associated with fractures

During the healing process:

1 Delayed union or non-union caused by infection, poor blood supply, interspersed fragments of tissue such as muscle, or movement of the fractured parts.
2 Malunion, rotation of a spiral fracture, or angulation of a transverse fracture.

Associated problems:

1 Soft tissue response: pain and gross oedema.
2 Tendon adhesion of the closely allied flexors and extensors.
3 Joint stiffness, particularly PIP joint flexion contracture.
4 Development of reflex sympathetic dystrophy.

Open reduction and fixation of fractures

See Figure 5.3.

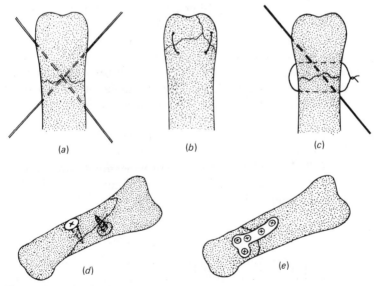

Figure 5.3 *Methods of internal fixation. (a) Crossed Kirschner wires. (b) Interosseous wiring. (c) Interosseous wiring combined with a Kirschner wire. (d) Cortical screws. (e) Compression plate. (From Opgrande and Westphal, 1980, by permission)*

Indications

1 Fractures that are unstable, inadequately reduced or compound (associated with an open wound).
2 Fractures that involve a joint surface, multiple fractures and fractures with bone loss.
3 Fractures where there is a need for early restoration of joint movement.

Techniques

1 Kirschner wires. In transverse fractures these are placed diagonally in opposite directions. In spiral fractures the wires are placed in parallel. It is important to make sure the Kirschner wires do not transfix the tendons over the fracture site and thus prevent the movement of joints on either side of the fracture.
2 Interosseous wire sutures can provide fracture apposition and compression in intra-articular fractures. It is sometimes difficult to achieve absolute stability because of the compressive forces across the joint.
3 The combination of a Kirschner wire and an interosseous wire is useful in transverse fractures of the phalanges or metacarpals. This technique provides stability as well as fracture compression and allows for early movements.
4 Cortical screws can provide excellent stability in spiral fractures. Two screws are placed at right angles to the shaft in different planes. Such fixation allows early movement and light functional activities.
5 Compression plates are useful for open reductions, e.g. transverse fractures of the metacarpals (Figure 5.4). They are rarely used for phalangeal fractures because too much stripping of periosteum and too much disturbance of tendon mechanism defeats the purpose of internal fixation.

Therapy for stable fractures

Metacarpal

Simple fractures of the metacarpals, e.g. the fifth metacarpal neck, are classified as stable fractures (Figure 5.5).

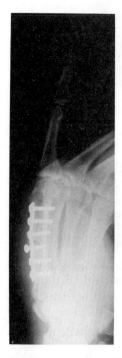

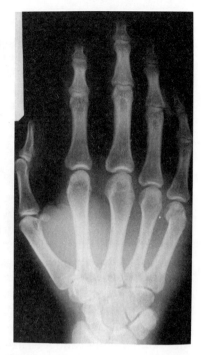

Figure 5.4 *Comminuted fracture of the fifth metacarpal shaft treated by a small compression plate and screws*

Figure 5.5 *Radiograph showing fracture of the neck of the fifth metacarpal*

Splintage

A short cock-up splint is used to support the wrist and aid reduction of oedema (Figure 5.6). The patient is instructed in shoulder exercises.

Treatment

Oedema is treated promptly with ice packs and elevation in a high sling and compression measures such as Tubigrip or 5 cm Coban wrap are also used.

With the wrist held extended, the patient practises gentle active MCP joint flexion within the limits of pain.

It is important to show the patient how to achieve effective MCP joint flexion in the first exercise session, as residual pain and oedema tend to result in flexion being initiated at the IP

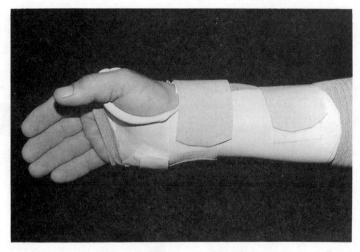

Figure 5.6   *Volar wrist extension splint is used to position and protect the hand following a stable fracture of the fifth metacarpal*

joints instead. If this tendency becomes a habit it will result in MCP joint stiffness and a weakened power grip.

It is not uncommon for a slight extension lag to occur at the level of the fracture site, i.e. at the MCP joint. This is managed by practising extrinsic extension exercises (performing MCP joint extension exercises with the IP joints held flexed); this problem is usually resolved within 3–6 weeks.

Once the fracture is healed, graded resisted exercises are added to the programme until full function is regained.

The splint is discarded after 1–2 weeks.

Phalangeal fractures

Therapy for stable phalangeal fractures is aimed at:

1 Prompt reduction of oedema and pain.
2 Institution of early active movements, i.e. within several days of injury.

Coban wrap (2.5 cm) is applied in a distal to proximal direction with even pressure.

The pressure of the Coban should not result in fingertip

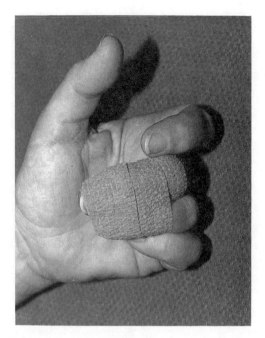

Figure 5.7   *Coban 2.5 cm is used to 'buddy-strap' the fractured digit to an adjacent one*

discoloration and the patient should not experience throbbing or numbness.

A short length of Coban can then be used to 'buddy-strap' the fractured digit to an adjacent finger (Figure 5.7).

Gentle active stabilized flexion and extension exercises of the IP joints can be carried out on an hourly basis. At this early stage, the patient may prefer to exercise with the buddy-strap in place as a means of providing extra support and pain relief.

When some fracture consolidation has occurred at 4–6 weeks, PIP joint flexion deformities which may have developed can be treated with a Capener splint (Figure 5.8).

Conversely, limitation of joint flexion can be treated with an IP joint flexion strap (Figure 5.9) or at a slightly earlier stage with the very gentle application of a crepe bandage which can hold the IP joints in a pain-free position of flexion for short periods, four to six times daily.

When there is evidence of good clinical and radiological union (approximately 6 weeks), graded resistance is added to the exer-

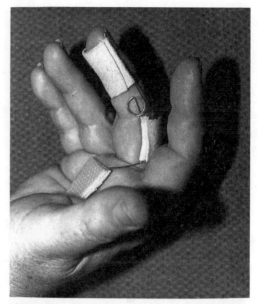

Figure 5.8 *Capener splint to treat a flexion deformity in the range of 30–45 degrees*

cises. If there is residual stiffness, passive joint mobilization techniques such as lateral and ventral gliding are used to increase flexion. These are followed by resisted exercises to maintain the increased joint range.

Therapy for unstable fractures following internal fixation

Metacarpal

1 Spiral fractured shaft.
2 Transverse fractured shaft.

Splintage after reduction and internal fixation

The hand is splinted in the POSI:

1 Wrist in comfortable extension.
2 MCP joints in maximum flexion.
3 IP joints in maximum extension.

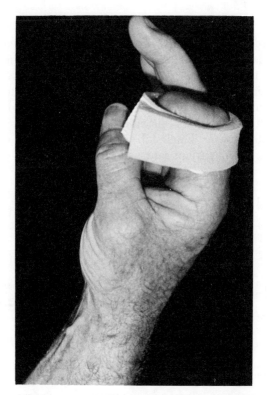

Figure 5.9 *Velfoam IP joint flexion strap for increasing flexion range*

Days 1–3

Dorsal oedema is significant following injury and surgery in this area. Ice packs are used 2-hourly with elevation of the hand. Shoulder and elbow exercises are practised.

Day 3–week 2

Providing the wound is not inflamed, active wrist flexion and extension exercises are started. The wrist is held extended and the MCP joints are actively flexed and extended. Holding the MCP joints in flexion, the PIP and DIP joints are flexed. All exercises are done within the limits of discomfort. Extrinsic extension exercises are practised to aid the specific glide of extensor tendons, which have a great tendency to form adhesions at the sites of fracture and operation.

Weeks 2–6

The sutures are removed and if the wound is healed, gentle lanolin massage is started. The splint may be shortened to a cock-up splint if oedema is controlled and pain has subsided. All exercises are continued, adding gentle resistance after the fourth week. Normal light use of the hand is encouraged as soon as possible after oedema has subsided.

A double leather fingerstall will lift a digit if extensor lag persists when the patient returns to work.

Proximal phalanx

See Figures 5.10 and 5.11a and b.

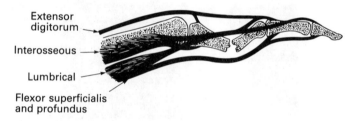

Figure 5.10   *Diagram of the muscle-tendon forces causing angulation of a fractured proximal phalanx. The extensor digitorum and lumbrical pull the head of the proximal phalanx dorsally, the interosseous pulls the base of the proximal phalanx volarly, and once angulation begins it is self-perpetuating*

Splintage

See Figure 5.12.

1 Wrist in comfortable extension.
2 MCP joints in maximum flexion.
3 IP joints in maximum extension.

Days 1–3

Oedema is treated as previously described and shoulder and elbow exercises are practised.

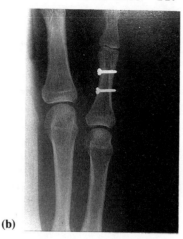

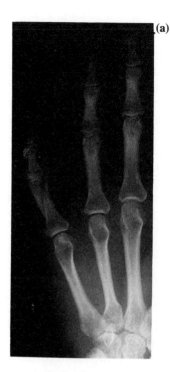

Figure 5.11 *(a) Spiral fracture of the proximal phalanx of the little finger. This fracture is potentially unstable and likely to rotate and shorten. (b) Treatment with small screws to prevent rotation and shortening*

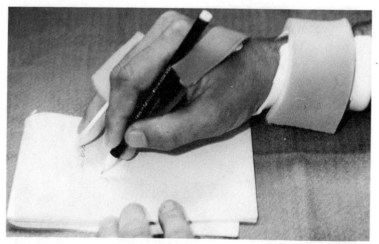

Figure 5.12 *Splint for immobilization following internal fixation of an unstable proximal phalangeal fracture of the little finger. Note the patient is able to use the radial three digits*

Day 3–week 2

All exercises are performed within the limits of discomfort. When the wound has settled, wrist movements and MCP flexion and extension exercises are started. Gentle stabilized PIP and DIP flexion are practised to promote specific glide of the FDP and the FDS, thus minimizing flexor tendon adhesion. It may be necessary to use sterile gloves if the wound is discharging slightly. To maintain finger mobility, gentle gross flexion is attempted. This may not be possible initially because of pain and oedema. The MCP joints are held in flexion and IP extension is practised (i.e. intrinsic extension) to minimize adhesion of the intrinsic extensor mechanisms over the dorsum of the fracture.

Weeks 2–6

The sutures are removed and lanolin massage is started if the wound is healed. The above exercises are continued, aiming at full flexion as soon as possible. Digital oedema is reduced and controlled by means of a Lycra fingerstall. The large splint is used for travelling and sleeping. The patient practises exercises 2-hourly depending on tissue reaction: if oedema increases then the exercise frequency is decreased. If there is tendon lag, i.e. inability

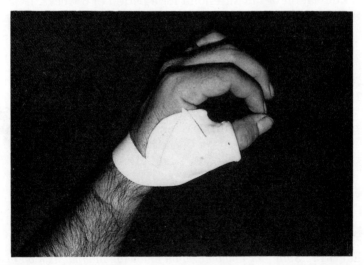

Figure 5.13 *Thumb post used to immobilize the MCP joint following injury to or repair of the ulnar collateral ligament*

to extend the IP joints fully and actively, a dorsal finger splint holding the PIP joint in extension is used in between exercise sessions. When there is evidence of union, graded resisted exercises and activities are commenced.

If the patient experiences difficulty in carrying out everyday activities because of a limited range of movement in the initial stages, then building up small handles, e.g. of cutlery and razor, aids the return of movement and function.

Common thumb injuries

Ulnar collateral ligament of the MCP joint

The mechanism of injury to this ligament involves falling onto the abducted thumb; this is an injury frequently sustained by skiers.

Sprain

Partial rupture of the ulnar collateral ligament is considerably more painful than complete rupture.

Treatment involves immobilization in a thumb post with slight ulnar deviation of the MCP joint for a period of 6 weeks. IP joint mobility is maintained during this time (Figure 5.13).

Complete rupture

Repair of the ligament is ideally performed within 7 days of injury. Following repair, the MCP joint can be held in extension by a K-wire for 2–3 weeks. A thumb post is used for immobilization and is worn for a further 4 weeks following K-wire removal.

Gentle active movements of the MCP joint are performed on an hourly basis following removal of the splint.

During the immobilization period, IP joint mobility is maintained.

If there is an associated avulsion fracture with displacement, surgical reduction/fixation is advised.

Bennett's fracture

This fracture is an intra-articular fracture of the base of the first

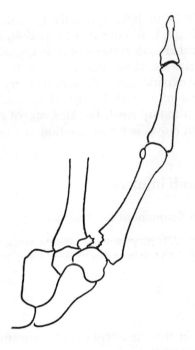

Figure 5.14   *Intra-articular fracture of the base of the first metacarpal (Bennett's fracture)*

metacarpal. It usually involves less than one-third of the articular surface and is accompanied by joint subluxation (Figure 5.14).

Unless the fracture is comminuted, the recommended treatment is open reduction and internal fixation using a cancellous screw.

This procedure facilitates early gentle active movement, usually 2–3 days after operation.

During the first 1 or 2 weeks after operation, the thumb can be protected with a thumb spica which is worn in between exercise sessions (Figure 5.15).

NB Because of the unique mobility and independence of the thumb, most shaft fractures of the first metacarpal can be treated conservatively, even in the presence of angulation or spiral deformity. Residual deformity is compensated for by the movements of the saddle-shaped first carpometacarpal (CMC) joint.

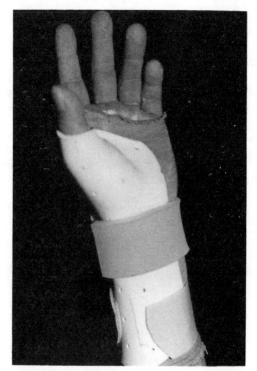

Figure 5.15 *Thumb spica used to protect the first CMC joint following internal fixation*

References and further reading

Barton, N. J. (ed.) (1988) *Fractures of the Hand and Wrist*, Churchill Livingstone, Edinburgh

James, J. I. P. (1970) Common, simple errors in the management of hand injuries. *Proceedings of the Royal Society of Medicine*, **63**, 69–71

Kalternborn, F. M. (1980) *Mobilization of Extremity Joints*, Olaf Norlis, Oslo

Maitland, G. D. (1977) *Peripheral Manipulation*, Butterworths, London

Milford, L. (1971) The hand. In *Campbell's Operative Orthopaedics*, 5th edn (ed. A. H. Crenshaw) C. V. Mosby, St Louis

Moberg, E. (1950) Use of traction treatment for fractures of phalanges and metacarpals. *Acta Chirurgica Scandinavica*, **99**, 341–352

Opgrande, J. D. and Westphal, S. A. (1980) Fractures of the hand. *Orthopaedic Clinics of North America*, **14**, 779–792

Opgrande, J. D. and Westphal, S. A. (1983) Fractures of the hand. *Orthopaedic Clinics of North America*, **14**, 779–792

Sandzén, S. C. Jr., Sigurd, C. (1986) *Atlas of Wrist and Hand Fractures*, 2nd edn, PSG Publishing, Massachusetts

Swanson, A. B. (1970) Fractures involving the digits of the hand. *Orthopaedic Clinics of North America*, **1**, 261–274

Wilson, R. L. and Carter, M. S. (1990) Management of hand fractures. In *Rehabilitation of the Hand: Surgery and Therapy*, 3rd edn (eds. J. M. Hunter, L. H. Schneider, E. J. Mackin *et al.*) C. V. Mosby, St Louis, pp. 295–303

Wright, T. A. (1968) Early mobilization in fractures of the metacarpals and phalanges. *Canadian Journal of Surgery*, **11**, 491–498

Wynn Parry, C. B. (1981) The stiff hand. In *Rehabilitation of the Hand*, Butterworths, London, pp. 234–248

6

Finger joint injuries

Anatomy

Finger joints consist of two cartilage-covered bone ends held together by a joint capsule. This capsule is strengthened on both sides by collateral ligaments and on the palmar surface by the palmar plate (Figure 6.1).

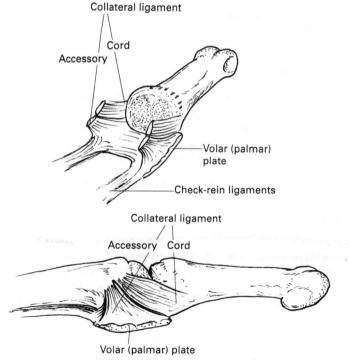

Figure 6.1 *Collateral ligament and volar (palmar) plate of the PIP joint*

The MCP joints readily stiffen in extension from fibrosis of the collateral ligaments. The IP joints readily stiffen in flexion from fibrosis of the palmar plate.

The injuries and treatment described here relate to the PIP joint.

Complications

1 Pain.
2 Oedema.
    (a) Acute: soft oedema that is able to be depressed by touch.
    (b) Chronic: tends to be brawny and unyielding.
3 Stiffness.
4 Flexion contracture.
5 Instability.

Aims of therapy

1 To reduce pain and oedema.
2 To regain range of movement.
3 To prevent a flexion contracture.

Classification

1 Sprain. Basically a soft tissue injury requiring conservative treatment.
2 Stable dislocation without ligament rupture.
3 Unstable dislocation with ligament rupture with or without an avulsion fracture. This injury requires surgical repair (Figure 6.2).

Sprain

A sprain is an injury to the structures of the joint, i.e. stretching or partial tearing of ligaments with no joint disruption.

Treatment should not be given until a radiograph has excluded a fracture or until examination (under a local anaesthetic, if necessary) has eliminated the possibility of ligament rupture.

Treatment

This is often a very painful injury with a gross oedematous

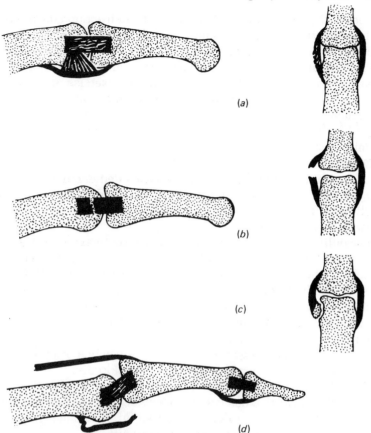

Figure 6.2 *Types of PIP joint injury. (a) Sprain of the collateral ligament system. (b) Rupture of the collateral ligament. (c) Rupture of the collateral ligament with an avulsion-type fracture. (d) Dorsal dislocation of the PIP joint with avulsion of the distal attachment of the palmar plate at the base of the middle phalanx*

response. Reduction of oedema generally has the effect of mini-mizing pain; oedema should therefore be treated promptly using ice massage followed by application of 2.5 cm Coban wrap.

To support the finger and protect it from re-injury, the digit can be 'buddy-strapped' to an adjacent digit with the Coban.

Alternatively, the finger can be immobilized for 3–5 days in a well-padded dorsal finger splint in a comfortable range of exten-sion until the initial discomfort has subsided.

Gentle, active stabilized IP flexion and extension exercises are usually commenced towards the end of the first week after injury. These exercises are performed on an hourly basis and sessions are kept short with five to ten movements, gradually increasing the number of movements as tolerance to exercise improves. Exercises should be carried out slowly and gently but in a sustained manner.

With any collateral ligament injury, the adjacent lateral bands of the extensor tendon or the oblique retinacular ligament may become adherent; to help prevent this adherence from becoming a contracture, intrinsic stretching is incorporated into the exercise programme. The intrinsic muscles are stretched by holding the MCP joints in the extended position while passively flexing the IP joints.

The oblique retinacular ligament is placed on maximum stretch by holding the PIP joint in full extension and asking the patient to actively flex the DIP joint. If this is not possible, the DIP joint should then be flexed passively in a gentle manner several times each hour. This procedure should always be carried out very slowly and the manoeuvre should not go beyond the point of pain.

Regaining flexion range can sometimes be as much of a problem as controlling the tendency toward flexion deformity.

Simple bandaging into flexion or the application of a flexion strap with minimal tension helps to overcome stiffness. These can be alternated with a dorsal finger splint or Capener (Figure 6.3a and b) which control the flexion deformity.

The patient is warned that ligaments are notoriously slow to heal and that symptoms of pain and stiffness may persist for many months.

Resisted exercises and activities are delayed until at least 6 weeks after injury.

Stable dislocation

See Figure 6.4a and b.

Joint alignment must be radiologically confirmed following reduction. The finger, together with an adjacent digit, is then splinted in the POSI with a thermoplastic splint.

The reasons for a large splint are:

1 There is usually considerable oedema which could be aggravated by the use of a finger splint.
2 PIP joint extension is best controlled with the MCP joints held in flexion.

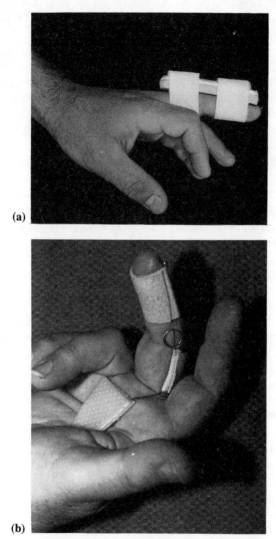

(a)

(b)

Figure 6.3 *(a) Dorsal finger extension splint can control a PIP flexion deformity where the joint can be passively extended to some degree with relative ease. (b) Capener is used to correct a PIP joint flexion deformity of 30–45 degrees and one that is resistant to passive extension*

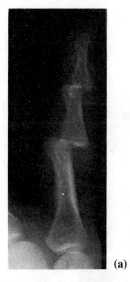
(a)

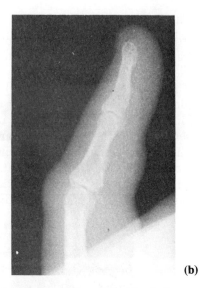
(b)

Figure 6.4   *(a) Radiograph showing dorsal dislocation of both IP joints. (b) Radiograph showing the reduced dislocations. Note that the lateral radiograph shows a small fracture of the base of the middle phalanx, possibly indicating rupture of the palmar plate*

Treatment

Treatment for a stable dislocation is very much the same as that described for sprains once the POSI splint is removed towards the end of the first week after injury.

After the fourth week, residual stiffness can be treated with passive joint mobilization in conjunction with the other therapy measures described earlier.

Traction, lateral gliding and dorsal or ventral gliding may be used according to which movement is limited.

Resisted exercises and activities are delayed until 8–10 weeks after injury.

Unstable dislocation

Dislocation of the PIP joint which has avulsed the palmar (volar) plate creates an unstable joint that tends to dislocate, resulting in a swan-neck deformity.

Surgery

Through a V-shaped volar approach, the flexor tendons are retracted and the palmar and lateral aspects of the PIP joint are dissected.

The distal end of the palmar plate is sutured to the base of the middle phalanx (Figure 6.5). This repair may need reinforcement, which is provided by using one of the slips of FDS, keeping its insertion at the middle phalanx, and suturing the proximal stump to the neck of the proximal phalanx.

To maintain the corrected position, a K-wire holds the joint in approximately 25 degrees of flexion and the hand is rested in a volar splint that extends to the tips of the fingers and maintains wrist extension.

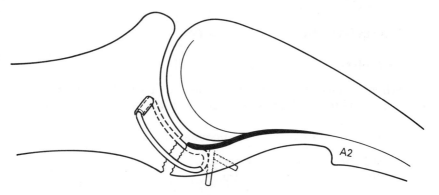

Figure 6.5 *Repair of palmar plate with pull-out wire suture*

Healing

The palmar plate takes 6–8 weeks to heal. The repair is protected by an internal splint, i.e. the K-wire, for about 3 weeks and then by a dorsal blocking finger splint, which maintains the 25 degrees of PIP joint flexion, for a further 3 weeks.

Postoperative management

If postoperative inflammation is severe, several days of rest are indicated and antibiotics may be given.

As soon as the inflammatory phase has subsided, gentle passive and active movements of the DIP joint are commenced. MCP joint mobility is maintained.

At 3 weeks, when the K-wire is removed, a dorsal PIP joint blocking splint maintaining 25 degrees of flexion, is applied to the finger. This splint is worn for 3 weeks and all exercises are carried out inside this splint.

Gentle unresisted active and passive PIP joint flexion exercises are commenced at this time.

Active extension of the PIP joint is commenced at the sixth week after operation. Passive PIP joint extension or extension splinting of this joint are rarely indicated as extension should only be achieved very slowly over the next 2–3 months.

Gentle resistance to flexion is applied from the sixth week.

Corrective surgical procedures

Arthrolysis

Where intensive conservative measures have failed to restore a functional range of movement, surgical freeing of the joint can be carried out.

This procedure is used most commonly for:

1 MCP joint extension contracture.
2 PIP joint flexion contracture.

There are two types of procedure:

1 Capsulotomy: division of the capsule or ligaments (collateral ligaments or palmar plate).
2 Capsulectomy: excision of the capsule.

Before the operation the therapist can provide the patient with detailed information regarding the post-surgical regimen.

Surgical technique

This operation is performed under selective peripheral nerve block. After adhesions have been freed, the patient actively moves the joint so that the degree of surgery necessary can be determined.

To maintain surgical gains, the joint is held by a Kirschner wire in the corrected position for 1–2 weeks. After removal of the wire, the joint is splinted appropriately, i.e. in MCP joint flexion following release of an MCP joint extension contracture, and in PIP joint extension following release of a PIP joint flexion contracture.

Postoperative management

Day 3–week 2

During Kirschner wire immobilization, unaffected joints are exercised to minimize tendon adhesion. Analgesia may be necessary before treatment for the first few days. The degree of pain and how long it persists varies considerably from patient to patient and for those patients who have had reflex sympathetic dystrophy (RSD) in the past, extra care must be taken.

Oedema control should be prompt and constant. High elevation is the primary treatment. Gentle compression bandaging with 5 cm Coban wrap for the dorsum of the hand or 2.5 cm Coban for the fingers can be used when the inflammatory response has subsided.

Week 2 onwards

Following removal of sutures, scar tissue is treated with lanolin massage and possibly ultrasound.

Active and passive flexion and extension exercises of the affected joint or joints are begun. Exercises are most effective when carried out often, i.e. hourly, for short sessions of five to ten repetitions. They should be performed slowly and in a sustained manner.

The patient must understand that exercise must be gentle enough to avoid tissue reaction but frequent and thorough enough to gently stretch adhesions.

When not exercising, the patient's hand is splinted in the position appropriate to maintaining and improving the position gained in surgery, i.e. in extension following release of a flexion contracture, and in flexion following release of an extension contracture.

Arthrodesis

Arthrodesis is fusion of a joint and is used because of instability or pain resulting from:

1 Joint disorder, e.g. osteoarthritis or rheumatoid arthritis, or a fracture/dislocation.
2 Tendon injury such as a ruptured flexor or extensor tendon.
3 Muscle-tendon palsy.

Surgery

All cartilage on each side of the joint is excised to enable exact bone apposition in the appropriate position, i.e. the position of function for that joint.

The fusion is held by a Kirschner wire, an encircling wire, a screw or a plate. The external K-wire is removed when there is radiological evidence of union, at approximately 8 weeks. Internal wires are not removed unless they are causing a problem.

Complications

1 Pain and oedema.
2 Stiffness of unaffected joints.
3 Non-union.

Healing

Bony union occurs in 6–12 weeks depending on the age and general condition of the patient and the condition of the bone.

Principles of aftercare

Stress on the fusion is avoided, but exercises of the joints proximal and distal to the fusion are commenced when postoperative inflammation has subsided.

References and further reading

Bennett, J. B. (1986) Joint injuries of the hand. In *Methods and Concepts in Hand Surgery* (eds N. Watson and R. J. Smith) Butterworth, London

Bowers, W. H. (1983) Management of small joint injuries in the hand. *Orthopaedic Clinics of North America*, **14**, 793–810

Bowers, W. H. (ed.) (1987) *The Interphalangeal Joints*, Hand and Upper Limb Series, Churchill Livingstone, Edinburgh

Dray, G. J. and Eaton, R. G. (1988) Dislocations and ligament injuries in the digits. In *Operative Hand Surgery*, vol. 1, 2nd edn (ed. D. P. Green) Churchill Livingstone, New York, p. 777

Eaton, R. G. (1971) *Joint Injuries in the Hand*, Charles C. Thomas, Illinois

Wilson, R. L. and Carter, M. S. (1990) Joint injuries in the hand: preservation of proximal interphalangeal joint function. In *Rehabilitation of the Hand: Surgery and Therapy*, 3rd edn (eds J. M. Hunter, L. H. Schneider, E. J. Mackin *et al.*) C. V. Mosby, St Louis, pp. 295–303

7

Flexible implant arthroplasty (metacarpophalangeal and proximal interphalangeal joints)

Flexible implants act as dynamic spacers, maintaining internal alignment of the reconstructed joint while early movement is begun. A successful arthroplasty should be stable, mobile, and painfree. The implant most commonly used is made of silicone elastomer.

Bone resection + Implant + Encapsulation = New joint (Swanson, 1973)

Indications and prerequisites

When the function of the MCP and/or PIP joints has been grossly impaired by rheumatoid, degenerative or traumatic arthritis, these joints can be replaced.

The successful outcome of this procedure depends on the patient's motivation and age.

Adequate soft tissue cover and an intact flexor and extensor muscle-tendon mechanism to motor the joint are important.

Surgical technique

Through a dorsal approach preserving the extensor and flexor tendon mechanisms, the head of the metacarpal or of the proximal

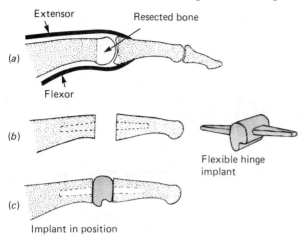

Figure 7.1 *Surgical technique for PIP joint Silastic arthroplasty. (a) Resection of damaged bone. (b) Reaming of bone. (c) Positioning the implant*

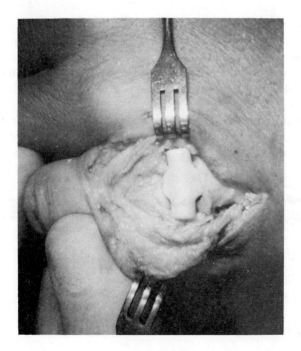

Figure 7.2 *Intraoperative photograph showing a Swanson Silastic implant with each stem in position. Note the retracted extensor apparatus*

phalanx is removed. The bone on either side of the joint is reamed to take the Silastic implant (Figures 7.1 and 7.2).

The collateral ligaments are divided proximally. This results in lateral instability until fibrous encapsulation occurs at around 3 months.

The capsuloligamentous structures around any flexible implant may be reconstructed to improve the stability and alignment of the implant (Figure 7.3).

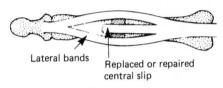

Lateral bands   Replaced or repaired central slip

Figure 7.3   *Reconstruction of the extensor apparatus*

Healing

Collagen gains strength rapidly during the first 3–4 weeks and continues to gain strength at a steady rate for 12 months or longer.

In the early stages of healing, the orientation and tension (tightness) of the developing capsule are very important. These are controlled by prolonged splinting and the institution of early exercises.

The deposition and remodelling of collagen around the implant (Figure 7.4) provide the reconstructed joint with a balance of stability and mobility.

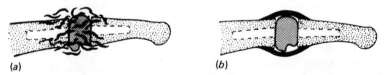

(a)   (b)

Figure 7.4   *Healing and reorganization ('training') of the joint capsule. (a) Untrained capsule. (b) Trained capsule*

Principles of management

1 Early active and passive movements.
2 Prolonged splinting.

3 Regular and long-term (2 years) follow-up to ensure maintenance of the range of movement.

If the desired range of movement has not been achieved
within the first 3–4 weeks, it is difficult to gain further
improvement.

Therapy programme for metacarpophalangeal implant arthroplasty

Complications

1 Oedema with or without inflammation.
2 Instability with lateral deviation and rotation.
3 Tendon adhesion leading to extensor lag.
4 Stiffness with limited flexion.
5 Fracture or dislocation.

Splintage

1 Wrist in comfortable extension.
2 MCP joints flexed to the midrange.
3 IP joints in extension.

Days 1–5

The hand is rested in the splint at all times, checking that the
bandage is holding the joints in proper alignment. Alignment is
assessed by looking at the patient's fingernail position in relation
to the line of the metacarpals.

Oedema is treated using:

1 Elevation of the hand in a sling or on pillows if the patient has
   shoulder or elbow problems.
2 Cold packs.
3 Rest.

Gentle elbow and shoulder exercises are practised.

Day 5–week 2

With the wrist held in slight extension, maximum active assisted
flexion and extension of the MCP joints of all fingers, in the pain-

free range, are commenced. All the fingers are moved simultaneously to maintain correct alignment, thus preventing the tendency to ulnar deviation.

These exercises are practised 5–10 times, every 2–3 hours. Once maximum flexion of the MCP joints is gained the IP joints are also flexed, aiming at gross flexion.

Particular attention should be given to flexion of the ulnar (ring and little finger) MCP joints. Full flexion of the index and middle fingers is less critical in grip function.

In attempting gross flexion there is a strong tendency to initiate flexion at the IP joints using the extrinsic flexors instead of using the intrinsic MCP joint flexors. This tendency must be corrected early and the patient taught to flex the MCP joints first, before closing the rest of the hand.

To promote effective MCP joint flexion it is helpful to immobilize the IP joints in extension by dorsal finger extension splints during exercise sessions.

Exercises are performed within the limits of discomfort.

Weeks 2–4

The sutures are removed. In the absence of inflammation, gentle lanolin massage is started. Effleurage assists the reduction of oedema around the joints.

The above exercise frequency is increased to 1–2 hourly sessions. If there is wound reaction, i.e. pain or swelling, the exercise programme is stepped down.

Extrinsic extension exercises are added to the exercise programme. These mobilize the extrinsic extensor tendons thus reducing the tendency to extensor lag.

When oedema and inflammation have subsided, and if there is a tendency to ulnar deviation, an outrigger splint is applied (Figure 7.5).

Outrigger position

The wrist is in slight extension. The splint extends just proximal to the MCP joints and the finger slings are placed on the proximal phalanges.

To prevent recurrent ulnar drift, the direction of pull on the digits should be towards the radial side.

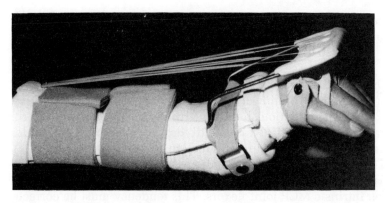

Figure 7.5 *Dorsal outrigger splint is used to control alignment after MCP joint arthroplasty*

MCP joint flexion can be practised against the gentle resistance of the elastic bands.

At 3 weeks there is often some degree of tightness of the dorsal capsule resulting in some limitation of MCP flexion. This tightness is overcome by the use of an MCP flexion splint. The outrigger and the MCP flexion splint are alternated according to need and progress. The splinting regimen for each patient is assessed regularly and modified accordingly.

During this first month, achievement of maximum MCP joint flexion is vital because it is difficult to gain a significant increase in the range of flexion after this time.

Weeks 4–8

The exercise regimen is maintained and the hand is used gently in light daily activities.

Modification of everyday utensils may be indicated, for instance padding of handles to aid grip.

Gentle resistive activities are introduced at 6 weeks.

Use of the MCP flexion splint is continued at night and intermittently during the day.

Because scars remain metabolically active structures for many months with a recurring tendency to tightening of the capsule, the MCP flexion splint regimen may need to be continued for a number of months.

Week 8 onwards

The hand is used for heavier activities and normal use is slowly resumed over the ensuing weeks.

The patient must understand that formal exercise may need to be practised for up to 1 year to gain the best possible result.

All splinting is discarded at week 12.

Therapy programme for proximal interphalangeal arthroplasty

Complications

1 Oedema with or without inflammation.
2 Instability with lateral deviation and rotation.
3 Recurring PIP flexion or extension contracture depending on which of these was present before surgery.
4 Fracture and/or dislocation.

The type of postoperative splinting and exercise programme depends on:

1 Whether the pre-existing contracture was in the extended or flexed position.
2 Whether extensor tendon reconstruction was necessary.

Therapy programme in the absence of extensor tendon reconstruction

Splintage

For pre-existing flexion contracture the hand is splinted in the POSI, i.e. with full IP extension.

For pre-existing extension contracture the hand is splinted as for flexor tendon repair, i.e. with the elastic band maintaining the PIP joint in some flexion.

Days 1–3

Oedema is treated with 2.5 cm Coban and elbow and shoulder exercises are practised.

Day 3–week 2

Gentle active flexion and extension exercises are begun. Initially 5–10 movements are practised 2–3 hourly, gradually increasing to 10–15 movements six times daily by the end of the second week.

To provide lateral stability, all fingers are exercised together.

Once oedema is controlled following flexion contracture release, a well-padded dorsal finger extension splint replaces the immediate postoperative splint. Following extension contracture release the postoperative splint can be replaced by a wrist strap to which the elastic band is attached.

Stabilized active flexion and extension exercises of the DIP joint are practised to promote glide of the flexor and extensor mechanisms.

Weeks 2–4

Individual stabilized active flexion of the PIP joint is started once there is some stability of the joint.

Intrinsic extension exercises combined with gentle passive extension of the PIP joint are also started.

Once the wound is fully healed, if there is residual oedema then a Lycra fingerstall is applied. The Lycra stall should have only slight tension to ensure ease of application. For stability, the digit can be 'buddy-strapped' to an adjacent finger during exercise.

Weeks 4–5

Gentle resistance is added to the exercise regimen and gradually upgraded during the following weeks.

Weeks 5–12

Gentle activity is commenced.

If full extension cannot be gained by means of a dorsal finger splint, an outrigger splint is applied.

As the extensor mechanism heals it tends to become tight, thereby preventing flexion. If this occurs, a PIP flexion splint is

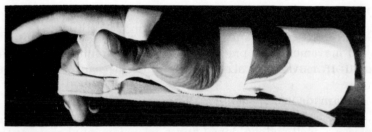

Figure 7.6 *PIP flexion splint used to overcome extensor tightness following PIP joint arthroplasty*

fitted and used intermittently during the day and at night (Figure 7.6). As with all splints, the tension and frequency of use are adjusted for each patient and monitored regularly.

Week 12 onwards

Normal activity may be resumed but, as with MCP arthroplasty, the exercise and splinting regimes need to be continued for many months to gain the optimum result.

Therapy programme in the presence of extensor tendon reconstruction

Active exercises are delayed for the first 10 days after operation.

Swan-neck deformity

Splintage

1 Wrist in slight extension.
2 MCP joints in flexion.
3 IP joint in 20 degrees flexion.

When postoperative oedema has subsided, the initial splint is replaced by a well-padded dorsal finger splint with the PIP joint held in 20 degrees flexion. The joint is splinted in this position to prevent the tendency to recurrence of hyperextension.

It may be necessary to wire the DIP joint in extension to maintain adequate correction of the deformity.

After the tenth day the exercises are practised as previously described for arthroplasty without tendon reconstruction.

Boutonnière deformity

Splintage

The hand is held in the POSI.

When postoperative oedema has subsided, the initial postoperative splint is replaced by a dorsal finger extension splint. The DIP joint is kept free to allow movement.

After the tenth day the previously described exercise regimen is followed. In between exercise sessions the digit is replaced in the finger extension splint to maintain correction. This splintage may need to be continued for 3–6 weeks depending on the degree of extension lag.

If the use of a PIP flexion splint is warranted, its application should be postponed until the seventh week after operation so as not to overstress the reconstructed extensor tendon mechanism.

References and further reading

Beckenbaugh, R. D. and Linscheid, R. L. (1988) Arthroplasty in the hand and wrist. In *Operative Hand Surgery*, vol. 1, 2nd edn (ed. D. P. Green) Churchill Livingstone, New York, pp. 167–214.

Madden, J. W., Arem, A. and De Vore, G. (1977) A rational postoperative management programme for metacarpophalangeal joint implant arthroplasty. *Journal of Hand Surgery*, **12**, 358–366

Shurr, D. G. (1986) The therapist's role in finger joint arthroplasty. In *Hand Rehabilitation* (ed. C. A. Moran) Churchill Livingstone, New York

Swanson, A. B. (1973) *Flexible Implant Resection Arthroplasty in the Hand and Extremities*, C. V. Mosby, St Louis

Swanson, A. B., de Groot Swanson, G., Leonard J. *et al.* (1990) Postoperative rehabilitation programmes in flexible implant arthroplasty of the digits. In *Rehabilitation of the Hand: Surgery and Therapy*, 3rd edn (eds J. M. Hunter, L. H. Schneider, E. J. Mackin *et al.*) C. V. Mosby, St Louis) pp. 912–928

8

Amputations (digital and partial hand)

Causes

Amputations may be carried out for congenital, traumatic or surgical reasons. The surgical indications for amputation include:

1 Irretrievable circulation.
2 Malignancy or severe infection.
3 Disuse resulting from persistent pain or joint stiffness which has been unresponsive to therapy or corrective surgery.

Classification

Amputations can involve:

1 Fingers: single or multiple digital amputation (Figure 8.1).
2 Thumb.
3 A combination of fingers and thumb. Radial or ulnar hemiamputation, or metacarpal amputation leading to a mitten hand (Figures 8.2–8.4).
4 The whole hand itself.

Surgical considerations for elective digital amputation

Requisites for a useful stump

1 Sufficient soft tissue cover.
2 Adequate length.
3 Sensibility.

Technique

This is shown in Figure 8.5.

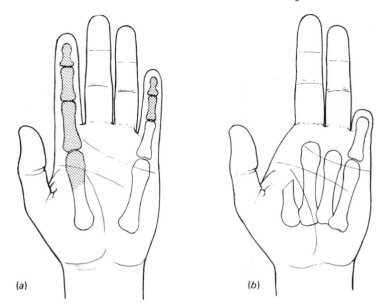

Figure 8.1 *Single digit amputations: ray amputation of the index finger and amputation through the PIP joint of the little finger*

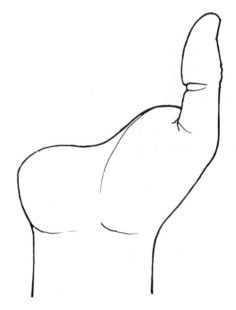

Figure 8.2 *The radial hand: loss of all four fingers*

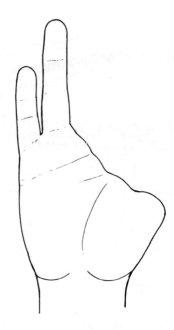

Figure 8.3   *The ulnar hand: loss of the radial three digits*

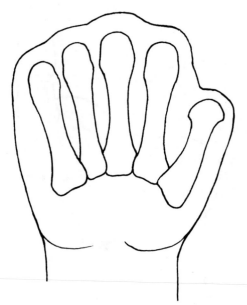

Figure 8.4   *The mitten hand: loss of all digits*

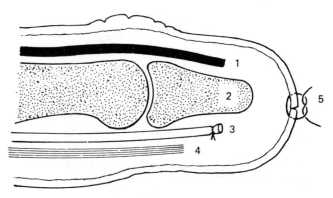

Figure 8.5   *Technique for amputation of a fingertip. 1 The extensor and flexor tendons are cut so that they retract from the stump. 2 The bone end is trimmed into a rounded stump. 3 The artery is dissected from the nerve and ligated. 4 The nerve is cut about 1 cm proximal to the stump. 5 The skin is closed loosely with fine sutures*

1 Skin flaps of sufficient size are raised to expose the underlying bone, flexor and extensor tendons, and neurovascular bundles.
2 If the amputation is through an IP joint, the articular cartilage is not removed, but the condyles and any rough projections of bone are nibbled away.
3 Flexor and extensor tendons are cut so that they lie away from the stump. If they are sutured over the stump, they interfere with the movements of the other fingers.
4 Digital nerves are dissected and cleanly divided about 1 cm proximal to the stump, so that any neuroma that forms is not at the scar line.
5 Skin is closed accurately and a non-adherent compression bandage is applied.
6 The wrist and the digit are splinted with a plaster slab and the hand is elevated for at least 48 h.

Problems and complications

These include:

1 Poor skin cover.
2 Poor circulation.
3 Neuroma.

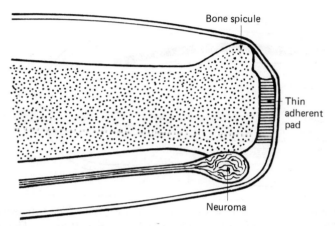

Figure 8.6 *Features of a problem stump showing a bone spicule, a thin adherent pad and a digital neuroma*

4 Stiff joints of the injured or adjacent digits.
5 Inadequate length.
6 Phantom pain.
7 Dystrophy (Figure 8.6).

Function and significance of respective digits

Thumb

The thumb is the most mobile and important digit of the hand and represents 40% of hand function. Maintenance of its length is vital.

The thumb, together with the index and middle fingers, is the primary digit for exploration.

Sensation to the thumb is as important to function as is movement, the hand being a sense organ.

The essentials of normal thumb function are:

1 Opposibility.
2 Stability.
3 Length.
4 Sensibility.

Index finger

The index finger represents 20% of hand function. It is fundamental to an effective pulp-to-pulp pinch grip, with or without the involvement of the middle finger.

Lateral pinch is the action of holding the thumb against the lateral side of the index finger, e.g. holding a saucer.

The index finger provides stability and balance in delicate everyday activities such as writing and drawing, and in the use of precision instruments.

Length is vital to the index finger. As the level of amputation in this digit approaches the PIP joint, pinch is transferred to the adjacent middle finger.

Middle finger

The middle finger represents 20% of hand function. It contributes to power grip, supports the index finger in pulp-to-pulp pinch grip, and provides a cupping action preventing small objects from falling through the hand when it is closed.

Amputation of the middle finger through the metacarpal results in loss of the stabilizing effect of the transverse metacarpal ligaments, causing the adjacent fingers to rotate towards the absent digit.

Ring finger

The ring finger represents 10% of hand function. Together with the little finger it is very important for power grip function. As is the case with the middle finger, metacarpal loss results in rotary deviation of the adjacent digits.

The ring finger also prevents small objects from falling through the closed hand (Figure 8.7).

This finger is important cosmetically as it is used for the purpose of wearing jewellery.

Little finger

The little finger represents 10% of hand function. It is an important digit in power grip, adding to the width of the grasp. It also helps in controlling fine movements in activities such as writing, because it extends the ulnar border of the palm.

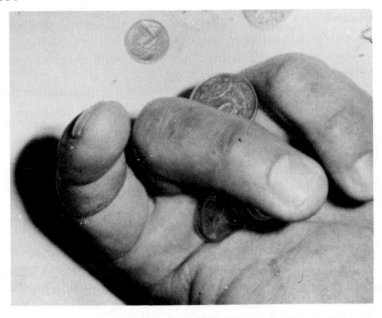

Figure 8.7 *Loss of the ring finger allows small objects to fall through*
the hand

In single digit amputations this is the least important digit
functionally.

Certain races keep the nail of the little finger long for cosmetic,
religious or practical reasons, e.g. for cleaning the ear (digit
auricularis).

Reconstruction

Assessment of suitability for surgery

The patient's suitability for reconstructive surgery is assessed in
terms of age, occupation, hand dominance and the ability to cope
with possibly numerous surgical procedures and lengthy aftercare
programmes.

A high level of motivation is essential to a successful outcome.

A thorough functional assessment is carried out to determine
the extent to which the patient's work, home and leisure activities
are limited.

Often, reconstruction or replantation are not worthwhile when the individual's particular physiological, psychological and economic states are considered.

Reconstructive surgery after amputation

This mostly means restoration of pincer grip function by:

1 Local rearrangement of hand remnants.
  (a) Deepening of the interdigital cleft, e.g. the thumb web, by Z-plasty lengthening of the skin and sliding the thenar muscle attachments down the shaft of the first metacarpal (Figure 8.8a and b).
  (b) Rotation osteotomy, in which the metacarpal is divided near its base and rotated or angulated so that the pulps of the digits oppose without tension.
  (c) Transfer of a digital stump, e.g. pollicization, when the metacarpal of the donor digit is divided and transferred to the recipient stump and internal fixation is used to stabilize the transferred digit.
2 Reconstruction of the thumb itself.
  (a) Replantation.
  (b) Toe transfer.
  (c) Bone graft and flap.
  (d) Bone lengthening.
3 Reconstruction of an opposition post.
  (a) Replantation.
  (b) Toe transfer.
  (c) Bone graft and flap.

Other reconstructive procedures include revision of scar by local or distant flaps.

Psychological aspects

Individual reaction to amputation is by no means always proportional to the extent of loss. One patient who has lost the tip of a single digit may be as traumatized as another who has lost several digits.

Religious and cultural factors are often highly significant in determining how someone reacts to loss of a part. In certain cultures, a man's worth in the eyes of the community and his self-esteem are based on his ability to provide for his wife and

(a)

(b)

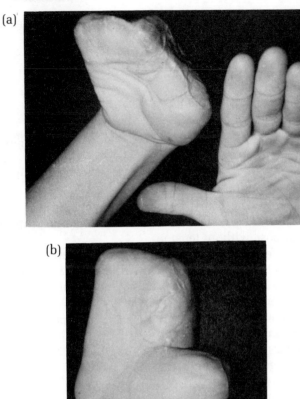

Figure 8.8 *(a) This 18-year-old's hand was caught in a circular saw, resulting in a mitten hand. (b) The recreation of a thumb web enabled this apprentice carpenter to complete his apprenticeship*

children, i.e. his breadwinner status. Loss of such status can have a devastating effect.

Whatever the psychological manifestation, it is important to afford it the same attention as the actual amputation, and referral to a social worker, psychologist or psychiatrist may be indicated.

Early postoperative therapy of digital amputations

The aim is to regain maximum movement and function of the remaining digits by exercise, desensitization techniques and early functional use.

Emotional support and constant reassurance are important aspects of the therapist's role during treatment.

Once satisfactory skin cover is achieved by surgery, and when stump circulation appears adequate, exercises are commenced (Figures 8.9 and 8.10).

Days 3–14

The wrist is splinted in a comfortable degree of extension.

1 Oedema is treated as previously described.
2 Stabilized active flexion and extension exercises are practised. These are followed by gross flexion and extension in the joints remaining.
3 Full range of movement is maintained at all upper limb joints.

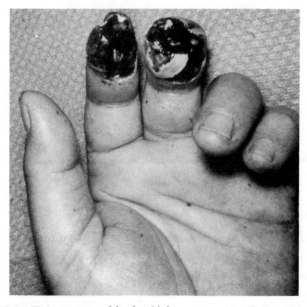

Figure 8.9 *This 45-year-old wharf labourer sustained a crushing injury resulting in amputation through the DIP joints of the index and middle fingers of his dominant hand*

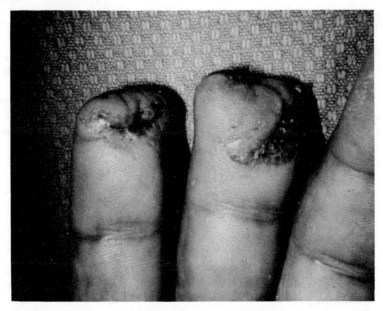

Figure 8.10 *Wound healing of 14 days following wound débridement and loose closure*

4 Early use of the remainder of the hand for easy everyday tasks is encouraged (Figure 8.11). This has the following advantages:
  (a) It helps prevent stiffness.
  (b) It discourages preoccupation with the injured hand.
  (c) It reassures the patient that, despite digital loss, the hand continues to be a useful functional unit and that he is bilateral.
  (d) It assists in desensitization of suture lines and grafted areas when these are healed.

Day 14 onwards

When the sutures have been removed or the graft site has healed:

1 The hand is given several Lux baths daily until the wound is clean.
2 Subaquatic pulsed ultrasound is commenced to assist desensitization.
3 Very gentle lanolin massage is begun to soften the scar line and as a means of initial desensitization (Figure 8.12). Care is taken

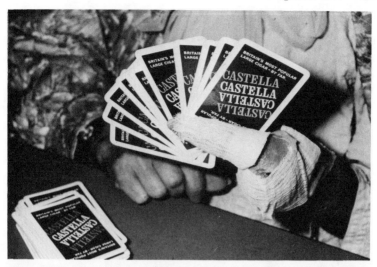

Figure 8.11 *Early pinch grip function was encouraged in this 50-year-old kitchen worker who lost the ulnar three digits as a result of severe burns*

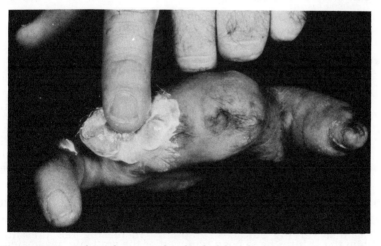

Figure 8.12 *When the wound is healed lanolin massage is carried out to soften the scar and desensitize the stump*

to avoid blistering the skin at this early stage. The patient is instructed to carry out massage six times daily for 5–10 minutes each session.

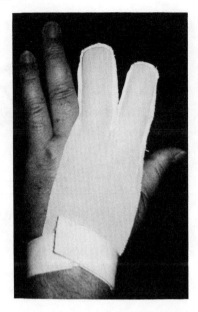

Figure 8.13   *Lycra fingerstalls assist stump shaping and reduce oedema*

4 Lycra fingerstall (Figure 8.13) is applied to:
  (a) Reduce residual oedema.
  (b) Assist stump shaping.
  (c) Assist in desensitization (by applying and removing the fingerstall).
5 The stump is stimulated with a variety of textures beginning with the softest and least irritating ones, e.g. cotton wool, and gradually increasing the coarseness of the texture as tolerance to touch improves (Figure 8.14a and b).
6 The stump is gently percussed by tapping it lightly with the fingers of the other hand and working up to tapping the stump against varying surfaces, gradually increasing the pressure. Graded activity also desensitizes the stump (Figure 8.15).
7 As tolerance to the above procedures increases, a vibrator can be used for the final stages of desensitization.
8 Graded activity programme is instituted to increase power in the remainder of the hand (Figure 8.16).
9 Snugly fitting soft leather fingerstall protects the stump for the first few weeks after return to work.

(a)

(b)

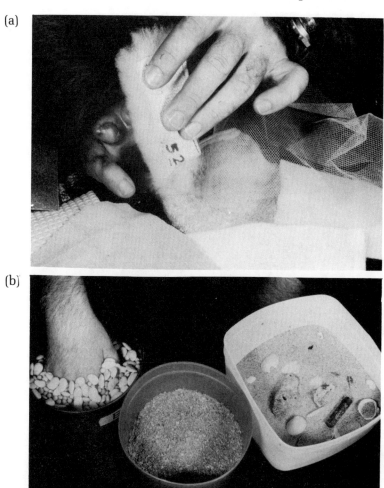

Figure 8.14 *(a) Graded textures are used to desensitize the stump. (b) Objects buried in containers filled with dried beans, sawdust, sand and so on, can be retrieved as a desensitization exercise*

Techniques for reduction of pain

If pain or hypersensitivity persists beyond 2–3 months after operation despite an active therapy programme, then the follow ing measures, used singly or in combination, may prove beneficial.

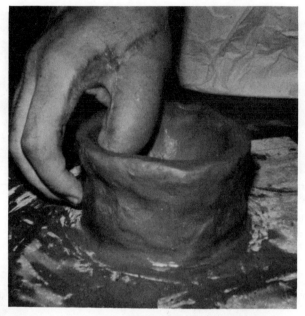

Figure 8.15   *Graded activity helps condition the stump*

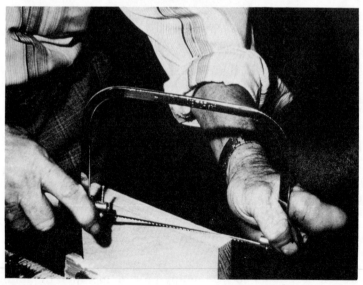

Figure 8.16   *Strength is gradually restored to the hand by way of various activities*

1 Transcutaneous electrical nerve stimulation (TENS). The pain relief response varies from patient to patient. Some patients experience prolonged relief for several hours by using TENS for only several minutes a day, while others need to use it constantly.

Some patients need to use the stimulator for only a few weeks for full efficacy, but it is more usual for pain relief to improve slowly over a period of several months.

The stimulator replaces the pain with a mild buzzing or tingling sensation. Some patients find this extremely unpleasant and TENS should be discontinued in these cases.

2 Local injection combined with massage and percussion techniques.

3 Further surgery for recurrent neuroma.

4 Protective padding. This has a cushioning effect and often affords a measure of relief for the problem of recurrent neuroma (Figure 8.17a and b). Padding can be used either as a preoperative measure or where repeated surgery has proved unsuccessful.

If all the above measures are unsuccessful, referral to a specialized pain clinic is usually indicated.

Activities of daily living assessment

The therapist assesses the patient's ability to perform everyday tasks, i.e. personal care, feeding and writing, and provides suitable aids, some of which may be required on a long-term or permanent basis (Figure 8.18).

These include:

1 A rocker knife which enables the patient to feed independently using one hand only.

2 Suction caps attached to a nailbrush to allow nail care of the remaining hand. The handle of the nail file needs to be enlarged to accommodate the suction caps.

3 Teaching the patient the one-handed method of tying shoe laces.

4 Early commencement of writing retraining where dominance must be changed.

Many patients are very adept in designing aids particular to their functional needs (Figure 8.19).

(a)

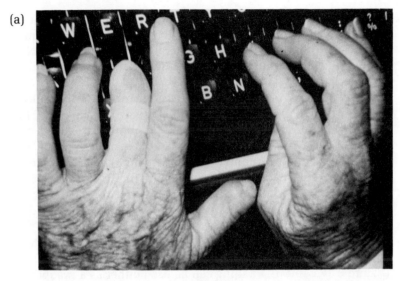

(b)

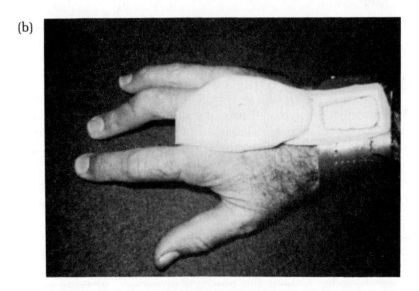

Figure 8.17 *(a) This secretary was able to resume work despite persistent sensitivity, by applying a rubber fingerstall over cotton padding. (b) Thick Velfoam padding enabled this railway shunter to return to work despite severe hypersensitivity as a result of recurrent neuromata*

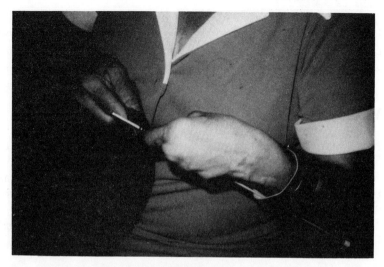

Figure 8.18 *A leather forearm cuff supports the knitting needle usually held by the middle, ring and little fingers*

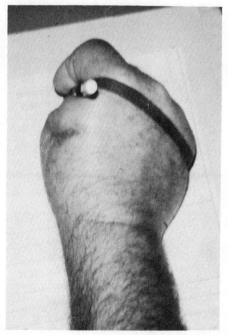

Figure 8.19 *While awaiting a thumb web reconstruction this 40-year-old engineer used a wide elastic band to stabilize his pen*

Ideally, aids should be kept to a minimum and used only as a last resort. They should be specifically tailored to the individual because two patients presenting with the same level of amputation do not necessarily have the same functional deficit.

Work assessment and retraining

In the latter stages of treatment the patient is assessed in terms of his or her ability to resume preinjury work.

Treatment activities should simulate work tasks as closely as possible within the confines of the therapeutic situation (Figure 8.20).

If there is any confusion regarding job requirements, a job visit is undertaken. This provides a realistic picture and allows

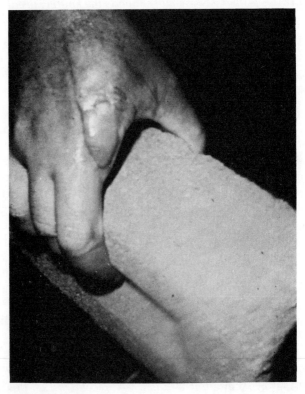

Figure 8.20   *Simulation of work tasks*

alternatîve solutions to be sought in the event that resumption of preinjury work is not possible.

Work retraining programmes are made available to those patients who do not have alternative skills.

Partial hand prostheses

Basic hand function includes:

1 Digital pinch (thumb opposed to fingers).
2 Palmar grasp (an object clasped securely in the palm of the hand).

It has the following requirements:

1 Durable skin cover with sensibility.
2 Mobile radial digit capable of contacting other elements of the hand (Figure 8.21a and b).
3 At least one stable ulnar digit within reach of the radial digit (Figure 8.22a and b).

Where reconstruction to provide the above is neither possible nor feasible owing to the patient's age or hand dominance, or to the long-term nature of reconstruction being impractical, a prosthetic aid for either function or cosmesis, or both, should be provided.

The cosmetic appearance of the hand is of major importance to many patients immediately following amputation, especially to women. Many demand immediate fitting of a cosmetic glove. It must be pointed out that the final fitting of any prosthetic device can only be made on to a stable desensitized stump (Figure 8.23).

It has been our experience that preoccupation with cosmesis lessens as patients become involved in their therapeutic programme and begin to use their hand again. They realize that the hand appears most normal when it is being used, with the result that many cosmetic gloves are actually rejected when they are finally fitted.

The most common and useful types of functional hand prostheses are those providing an opposition bar against 'which the remaining digit or digits, be they ulnar or radial, can be opposed.

(a)

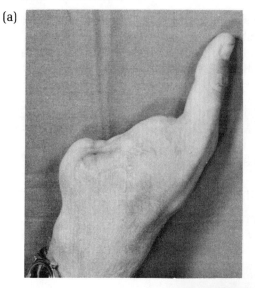

(b)

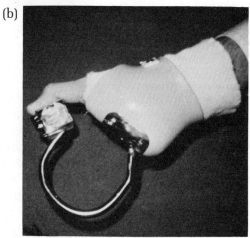

Figure 8.21   *(a) This 18-year-old student draughtsman lost all his fingers in a mincing machine while working at his part-time job. (b) A partial hand prosthesis with an opposition bar providing effective pincer function*

(a)   (b)

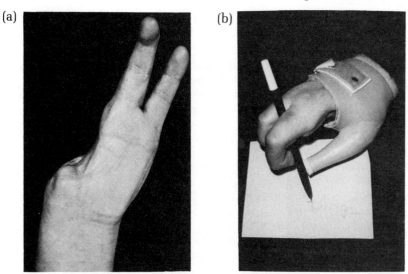

Figure 8.22 *(a) This young Lebanese process worker lost her radial three digits in a press at a car assembly plant. (b) A thumb opposition post made pinch grip possible*

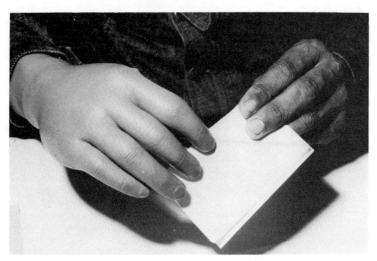

Figure 8.23 *In public some patients prefer to wear a cosmetic prosthesis*

References and further reading

Hunter, J. M., Schneider, L. H., Mackin, E. J. *et al.* (eds) (1990) Amputation and prosthetics. In *Rehabilitation of the Hand: Surgery and Therapy*, 3rd edn, C. V. Mosby, St Louis, pp. 997–1091

Louis, D. S. (1988) Amputations. In *Operative Hand Surgery*, vol. 1, 2nd edn (ed. D. P. Green) Churchill Livingstone, New York, pp. 01–120

Sheahy, C. W. and Maurer, D. (1974) Transcutaneous nerve stimulation for the relief of pain. *Surgical Neurology*, **2**, 45–47

Swanson, A. B. (1964) Levels of amputation of fingers and hand – considerations for treatment. *Surgical Clinics of North America*, **44**, 1115

Tupper, J. W. and Booth, D. M. (1976) Treatment of painful neuromas of sensory nerves in the hand: a comparison of traditional and newer methods. *Journal of Hand Surgery*, **1**, 144–151

Wilson, R. L. and Carter-Wilson, M. S. (1983) Rehabilitation after amputations in the hand. *Orthopaedic Clinic of North America*, **14**, 851–872

Wynn Parry, C. B. (1981) The stiff hand. In *Rehabilitation of the Hand*, Butterworths, London, pp. 285–296

9

Dupuytren's contracture

In Dupuytren's contracture, first described by Guillaume Dupuytren in 1831, there is fibrosis and shortening of the palmar aponeurosis leading mainly to a flexion contracture of the digital joints and often to an adduction soft tissue contracture (Figure 9.1).

Dupuytren's contracture involves primarily the longitudinal bands of the palmar aponeurosis, the vertical extensions of the fascia of the skin and the oblique and horizontal fascia of the interdigital webs.

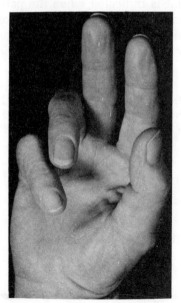

Figure 9.1 *Advanced Dupuytren's contracture with marked flexion deformities of the ring and little fingers*

This condition, of unknown aetiology, primarily affects Caucasian males and is rare among Oriental and Black races.

There is a positive family history in 25% of cases. Although Dupuytren's contracture occurs mainly in manual workers, it is also seen in sedentary workers. It has a higher incidence among alcoholics, diabetics and epileptics.

The average age of onset in men is about 48 years, while in women it is 59 years. Although the disease appears later in women and is usually less severe, the prevalence of reflex sympathetic dystrophy following surgery is twice as common in women. The overall incidence of this complication is approximately 4%.

Most patients with Dupuytren's disease have involvement of the ring and little fingers. If the disease is also present on the radial aspect of the hand, it is often more aggressive and difficult to treat.

Indications for surgery

Operative treatment is indicated when the palmar fascial bands cause a flexion contracture of the MCP or PIP joints or adduction contracture of the thumb or other interdigital webs.

The longer the contracture is present, the more difficult it is to correct.

The MCP joint can be readily released at any stage of the contracture, whereas release of an established PIP joint contracture is less predictable. For this reason, it is better to operate early when the PIP joint is involved.

Because of the potential incidence of a number of complications (e.g. haematoma, ischaemia and infection), it is prudent to inform the patient of their possible occurrence.

Types of operative treatment

Fasciotomy

This is simple division of the contracting band (Figure 9.2). The procedure is suitable for older patients because it provides a good early result; there is, however, some recurrence.

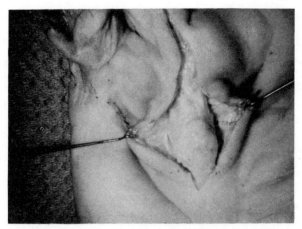

Figure 9.2 *Operative view showing a large Dupuytren's nodule and bands*

Fasciectomy

1 Radical (extensive resection of the entire aponeurosis). This procedure carries a risk of wound complications, such as haematoma or skin sloughing.
2 Local or regional. This gives the best overall result with the lowest morbidity (Figure 9.3).

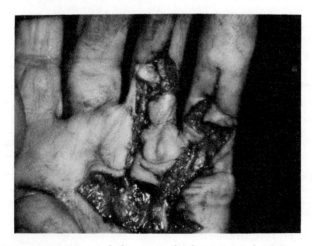

Figure 9.3 *Appearance of the wound after removal of Dupuytren's tissue by local fasciectomy*

Skin cover after fasciectomy can be obtained by:

1 Z-plasty or local flap repair.
2 Skin grafting in patients with recurrent disease, involved skin or insufficient skin for Z-plasty.
3 Open wound technique. The transverse wound of the palm or digit is left open to heal spontaneously (Figure 9.4). Early exercises can begin without the risk of haematoma or infection. Wound healing, which occurs by marginal epithelialization, is usually complete within 4–6 weeks. Betadine-soaked gauze used over the wound, hastens healing significantly.

Salvage procedures

1 Joint fusion.
2 Amputation with the use of filleted skin to close the palm defect.

Complications of healing

A combination of the following factors predisposes to wound and overall hand complications:

1 Older age.
2 Alcoholism and diabetes.
3 The surgical raising of extensive thin skin flaps.
4 Involvement of the skin in the disease process.
5 Extensive dissection involving the blood supply to the skin and deeper structures.
6 Excision of scar tissue on the flexor tendon sheath and IP joints.

Complications include:

1 Haematoma.
2 Oedema.
3 Infection.
4 Ischaemia and skin necrosis.
5 Tendon adhesions.
6 Joint adhesions and stiffness.
7 Palmar fasciitis.
8 Hypertrophic and contracting scar.
9 Nerve/artery damage.

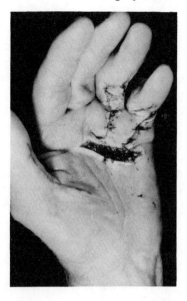

Figure 9.4 *Appearance of the hand following fasciectomy using Z-plasties in the fingers and the open palm technique (healing by secondary intention)*

10 Slow healing of the operative wound owing to poor circulation following months or years of fibrosis.
11 Reflex sympathetic dystrophy.

Fasciotomy

Postoperative management

Days 1–3

Splintage

1 Wrist in comfortable position.
2 MCP and IP joints in comfortable extension to maintain surgical gains.

Oedema is treated. Particular attention should be given to shoulder movements because most patients are in the older age group and the possibility of shoulder stiffness is therefore greater.

Days 3–7

Active wrist exercises are started, these being followed by finger exercises.

Stabilized active PIP and DIP flexion and extension exercises are practised to minimize tendon adhesions.

Gentle passive and active extension exercises are begun.

Days 7–14

Lux baths are given twice daily and continued until the wound is completely healed. These baths aid the removal of any devitalized tissue (eschar) and the warmth facilitates movement.

Day 14 onwards

Lanolin massage is started once the wound has healed. All exercises are continued, aiming at maximum extension and the regaining of full flexion.

Fasciectomy

Principles of postoperative management

1 Early diagnosis and prevention of wound complications, (e.g. removal of sutures from any area of skin with poor circulation) and prompt treatment of oedema.
2 Maintaining correction of the flexion deformity by appropriate splintage.
3 Regaining full flexion and grip strength.

Fasciectomy involves greater dissection of tissue within the hand; the potential postoperative scarring is therefore increased and particular attention must be given to reducing the tethering effects of the scar tissue by way of massage, exercise and splintage, for instance with a volar pan stretch splint or outrigger.

Day 3 – the onset of wound healing in the absence of grafting.

If there are skin grafts, exercise is delayed for approximately 7–10 days. Grafts are monitored carefully for vascularity during early healing.

1 Therapy is begun with gentle active wrist movements followed

by individual stabilized active PIP and DIP flexion exercises. These are performed 2–3-hourly with five to ten movements of each joint at each session.

For exercises to be carried out effectively, dressings should be kept to a minimum so that they do not impede movement.

2 Holding the wrist in extension, intrinsic MCP flexion (i.e. with the IP joints in extension) is practised. This is followed by gross flexion exercises of all three finger joints, the aim being to regain a full fist.

3 Active finger flexion is performed. This is followed by gentle passive extension, taking care not to overstress the wound.

4 The patient should practise opposition of the thumb to all the digits, and abduction/adduction of the fingers and thumb.

NB The appearance and condition of the hand is monitored closely during the first few weeks after operation as changes in circulation and oedema can occur quite markedly within the space of a few days.

The therapist should remain alert to oedema and stiffness which is accompanied by exaggerated pain as this may be heralding the onset of reflex sympathetic dystrophy.

At wound healing

1 The above exercise programme is continued.

2 Scar tissue is treated using:

(a) Subaquatic pulsed ultrasound.

(b) Intensive lanolin massage (where there have been skin grafts, massage is performed lightly to avoid blistering).

(c) To reduce very dense scarring, pressure is applied by means of a silicone elastomer mould worn beneath a Lycra pressure garment (Figure 9.5). These moulds are renewed every few days in accordance with changes in scar contour and are abandoned when the desired result has been achieved. For preparation of moulds using 382 Medical Grade Elastomer, the therapist should refer to the Dow Corning literature which accompanies the product.

3 Oedema in some cases is slow to resolve. A Lycra pressure garment is effective in its reduction (Figure 9.6).

4 Desensitization: sensitive scars are treated with gentle massage, pulsed ultrasound, gentle tapping and stimulation with a

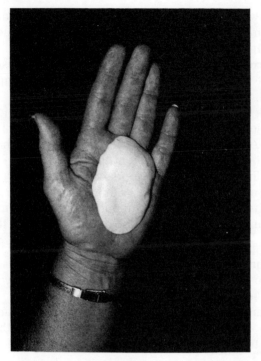

Figure 9.5 *Application of serial silicone elastomer moulds aids in the reduction of dense raised scar tissue. These moulds are worn beneath the pressure of a bandage or Lycra glove*

variety of textures, beginning with the least irritating, e.g. cotton wool and progressing gradually to coarser textures.

Where there are sensory changes (be they transient or permanent), the patient is given advice regarding protection from injury to anaesthetic areas.

5 The tendency for recurring flexion deformity is managed by:

(a) Gentle passive extension exercises.

(b) Application of a volar pan splint (Figure 9.7) which is worn intermittently throughout the day and all night. A wide, well-padded Velcro strap exerts gentle pressure over the dorsum of the PIP and/or MCP joints.

(c) A dynamic outrigger is indicated where there is a strong tendency for recurrence of the flexion deformity (Figure 9.8).

Owing to compromised vascularity and/or sensation, extra

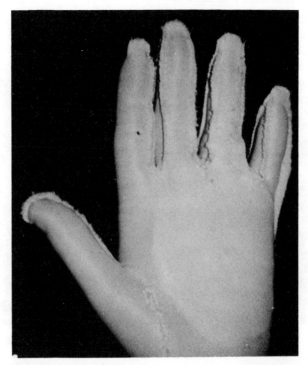

Figure 9.6 *Hand oedema that is slow to resolve is controlled by a Lycra pressure glove. Note the silicone elastomer mould being worn under the glove*

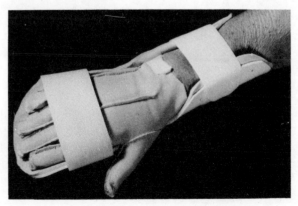

Figure 9.7 *Volar plan splint maintains surgical correction of the flexion deformity. The application of a wide well-padded Velcro strap provides a gentle extension force*

care must be taken during splint application. NB Extension splintage is often continued at night for 6 months or longer after the operation.

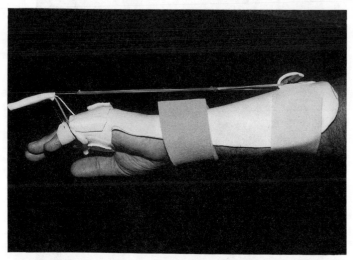

Figure 9.8   *Where there is a strong tendency for recurrence of the deformity after surgery, a dynamic outrigger splint is indicated*

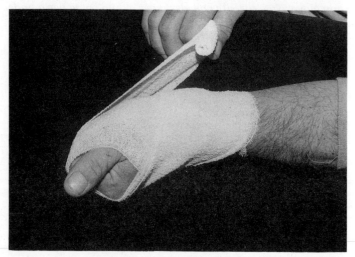

Figure 9.9   *Bandaging the fingers into flexion using a wide crepe bandage helps in regaining flexion range. Note that the wrist is in extension to facilitate finger flexion*

6 If there is difficulty in regaining flexion, this may be encouraged by bandaging the hand into flexion using a wide crepe bandage (Figure 9.9). This position is maintained for 15–20 minutes, five or six times daily.

The efficacy of this procedure is enhanced if heat (by way of wax, water or Fluidotherapy) is used simultaneously.

These sessions are followed immediately by concentrated active flexion exercises to capitalize on the increased flexibility of the joints.

When mid-range flexion has been achieved, the bandaging technique is replaced with a flexion strap made of neoprene or Velfoam to exert greater pressure over the IP joints (Figure 9.10).

It is important to strike a balance between maintaining extension and regaining maximum flexion. It takes some patients many months to regain an acceptable flexion range. This applies particularly to patients who have degenerative joint changes.

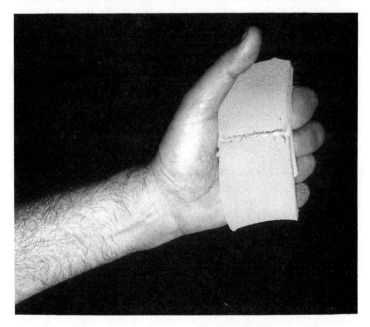

Figure 9.10 *Flexion strap applied to help regain further flexion once mid-range flexion has been achieved*

7 Light activity is begun as soon as the wound is healed. Enlargement of the handles of everyday utensils assists function until flexion range improves.

References and further reading

Fietti, V. G. and Mackin, E. J. (1990) Open-palm technique in Dupuytren's disease. In *Rehabilitation of the Hand: Surgery and Therapy*, 3rd edn (eds J. M. Hunter, L. H. Schneider, E. J. Mackin *et al.*) C. V. Mosby, St Louis, pp. 873–882

Hueston, J. T. (1963) *Dupuytren's Contracture*, Churchill Livingstone, Edinburgh

MacCallum, P. and Hueston, J. T. (1962) The pathology of Dupuytren's contracture. *Australian and New Zealand Journal of Surgery*, **31**, 241

McCash, C. R. (1964) The open palm technique in Dupuytren's contracture. *British Journal of Plastic Surgery*, **17**, 271

McFarlane, R. M. (1988) Dupuytren's contracture. In *Operative Hand Surgery*, vol. 1, 2nd edn (ed. D. P. Green) Churchill Livingstone, New York, pp. 553–590

McFarlane, R. M. and Albion, U. (1990) Dupuytren's disease. In *Rehabilitation of the Hand: Surgery and Therapy*, 3rd edn. (eds J. M. Hunter, L. H. Schneider, E. Mackin *et al.*) C. V. Mosby, St Louis, pp. 867–872

McFarlane, R. M., McGrouther, D. A. and Flint, M. H. (eds) (1990) *Dupuytren's Disease*, Churchill Livingstone, Edinburgh

Wynn Parry, C. B. (1981) The stiff hand. In *Rehabilitation of the Hand*, Butterworths, London, pp. 251–254

10

Crushed hand

Treatment of a patient with a crush injury can last for many months. Numerous reconstructive procedures may be necessary and each of these is invariably followed by several weeks or months of intensive therapy; patient motivation is therefore vital. To maintain this motivation the patient must understand the implications of the injury and the reasons for the various treatments. In other words, patient education is an important aspect of treatment. Only in this way will the patient feel that he is an important member of the team with increasing responsibility for his own aftercare.

Although the tissues involved, skin, tendons, blood vessels, nerves and bones (fractures and/or dislocations), and the degree of injury vary from one patient to the next, the principles of treatment remain the same: uncomplicated wound healing followed by early active movement.

The primary medical and surgical management to a large extent determines the ultimate outcome of hand function. These injuries warrant specialist care and patients should be transferred to a specialized hand unit. The only real emergency arises from vascular injury associated with ischaemia, the signs of which include:

1 Persistent throbbing pain.
2 Pallor.
3 Absent pulse.
4 Paraesthesia.

This emergency requires surgery in the form of decompression by fasciotomy and/or vessel repair.

Prevention of infection is of paramount importance. It may involve:

1 Appropriate antibiotics and tetanus immunization.
2 Wound debridement for removal of foreign material and devitalized tissue. This may need to be performed in several stages.

Depending on the degree of tissue loss, a skin graft or flap may be necessary to protect exposed tendons, nerves and bone. Where a skin graft or flap is not indicated, wounds are left unsutured and allowed to heal by secondary intention.

When there are fractures and/or dislocations in addition to significant soft tissue injury, management of these is of secondary importance. However, if there is circulatory embarrassment, gentle alignment of the finger aids circulation. The hand should be splinted in a position as close as possible to the POSI (see Figure 0.1).

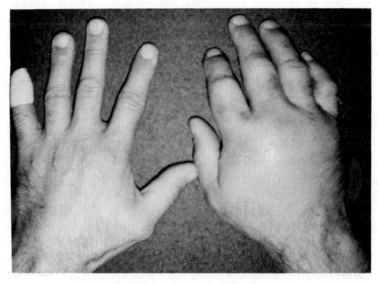

Figure 10.1 *Gross soft tissue reaction (oedema) following a crushing injury by a metal container*

Therapeutic mangement

The severity of the injury and the extent of individual tissue reaction dictate the timing of the various treatment methods used. These methods, however, vary very little from one patient to the next.

Oedema

The major complication common to crush injuries is gross oedema resulting in fibrosis and adhesion formation (Figures 10.1 and 10.2). Adhesions tend to form between tendon and skin, tendon and tendon sheath, tendon and bone, and in and around joints.

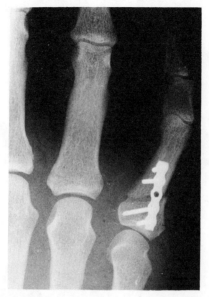

Figure 10.2 *Skeletal damage (fracture of the proximal phalanx) is relatively minor, but note the gross soft tissue reaction in Figure 10.1*

Oedema is controlled by:

1 Constant high elevation of the hand on pillows. This is preferable to a bedside sling which can have a constrictive effect on circulation at the elbow.
2 Cold therapy with ice packs (Figure 10.3).
3 Intermittent pressure as soon as the wounds are healed. The pressure unit (this device is not used in the presence of inflammation or infection) is applied in elevation for half-an-hour twice daily (Figure 10.4). The cycling phase is 5 s on, 5 s off, using a pressure of 20–40 mmHg.
4 Early active movement and light unresisted selfcare activities.
5 A Lycra pressure glove. The resolution of oedema following

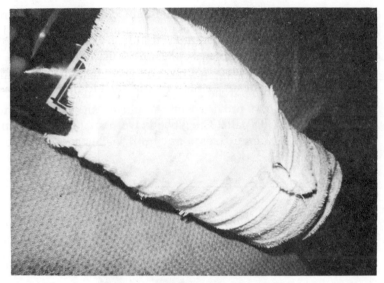

Figure 10.3 *Constant elevation and cold therapy aid reduction of oedema and pain*

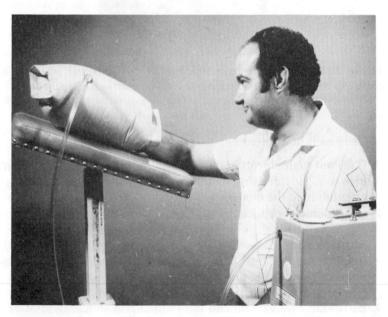

Figure 10.4 *At wound healing, intermittent pressure treatment is begun*

pressure treatment is effectively maintained by a Lycra pressure glove (Figure 10.5). As for pressure treatment, the garment is only applied over healed wounds and is contraindicated in the presence of inflammation or infection. If swelling is confined to the dorsum of the hand, the fingers may remain free from the level of the PIP joints if the glove is custom-made.

The firm support provided by the glove can also have the effect of alleviating pain. The glove is worn at all times except during formal therapy sessions, until oedema is resolved (Figure 10.6).

Pain

Pain is a significant factor following a crush injury and adequate analgesia before treatment enables effective exercise and engenders patient confidence. Ice and intermittent pressure treatment also help in pain reduction.

Stiffness

In the presence of uncomplicated wound closure, gentle active exercise can begin 2–3 days after the injury. These movements should be performed within the limits of pain.

Where skin grafting has been necessary, movements are delayed for approximately 7–10 days.

Movements should be carried out in a systematic fashion so that the patient is not observed to be merely wriggling the fingers. Gentle active stabilized flexion and extension exercises should be carried out at each finger joint in turn.

The patient tends to fatigue quickly at this early stage, so two or three short exercise sessions per day suffice during the first few days. The number of treatments and the treatment time can be gradually increased commensurate with improvement.

Restoration of MCP flexion is important and intrinsic flexion (that is with the IP joints held extended) should precede fist-making, with flexion at all three finger joints.

In between exercise sessions the hand is splinted in the POSI. This position may need to be modified owing to the presence of dorsal hand oedema.

To aid increase in joint range of movement, passive joint mobilization may be used as an adjunct to active exercise. For example to increase MCP flexion, the metacarpal is stabilized

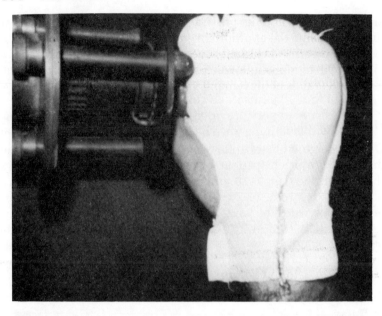

Figure 10.5 *Oedema reduction is maintained by a Lycra pressure garment worn during activity*

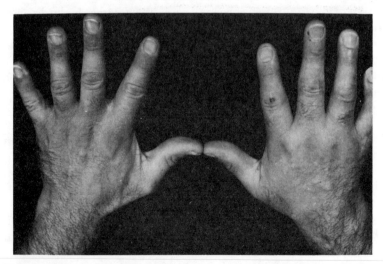

Figure 10.6 *Soft tissue reaction was almost completely resolved at 8 weeks and the full range of flexion and extension almost completely restored*

close to the joint and the proximal phalanx is mobilized in a volar direction, using the appropriate grade of mobilization.

Where possible, i.e. in the absence of unstable fractures, passive joint mobilization is followed by resisted exercise to maintain the gain in the range of movement.

Home programme

On discharge from hospital a suitable exercise programme is designed for each patient. Exercises are practised regularly throughout the day: 5–10 min of exercise every 1–2 h is far more beneficial than one or two lengthy sessions when the patient tends to overwork the joints and aggravate pain and oedema.

Without the continuity of a home programme, the therapist's treatment is futile.

Contracture

A number of patients, despite all preventative measures, develop some degree of stiffness or contracture (Figure 10.7).

Because release is as important as grasp in hand function,

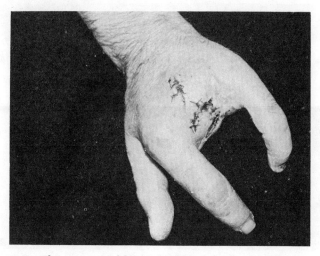

Figure 10.7 *This 43-year-old man had his left (dominant) hand caught in a garbage compactor. Poor circulation and Pseudomonas infection resulted in amputation of the middle and ring fingers at metacarpal level*

splinting in extension and in flexion may be balanced (Figures 10.8 and 10.9). For instance, an outrigger splint or joint jacks (Figure 10.10) to overcome PIP flexion contractures may need to be alternated with a PIP flexion splint to overcome a limited PIP flexion range (Figure 10.1.).

Owing to dorsal oedema, contracture of the MCP joints in extension is a common problem. This should be treated with an MCP flexion splint (Figure 10.8).

A thumb outrigger or serially applied C-splints will correct a tightly adducted thumb (Figure 10.12).

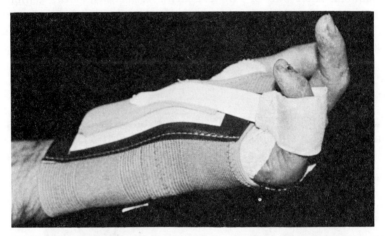

Figure 10.8 *Initially, limitation of flexion of the fifth metacarpal joint was overcome by an MCP flexion splint*

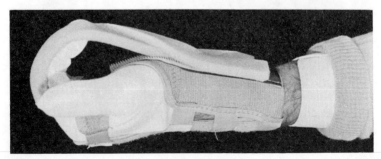

Figure 10.9 *Restricted flexion of the IP joints was treated with an IP flexion splint. This was alternated with the MCP flexion splint and finger extension splints*

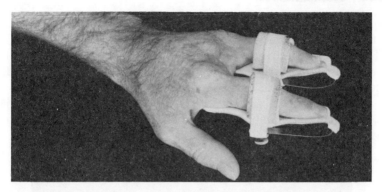

Figure 10.10 *PIP flexion contractures of 35 degrees in the remaining digits were treated with commercially available joint jacks*

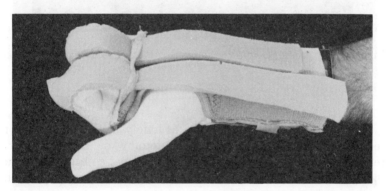

Figure 10.11 *Final degrees of passive flexion were achieved by the addition of a palmar band under which the flexion straps were threaded*

Weakness

To help restore strength to pinch grip and power grasp, a graded activity programme is instituted when resisted active exercises are commenced.

Grip measurements together with measurements of joint range are recorded on a regular basis to determine progress.

There may be phases when improvement reaches a plateau. At these times measurements are carried out less frequently so that the patient does not become despondent during this temporary cessation of progress.

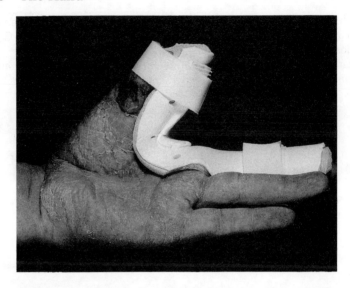

Figure 10.12   *Serial C-splints can be used to treat a contracted first web space*

Reconstructive procedures such as tenolysis, two-stage tendon reconstruction, joint release (capsulotomy or capsulectomy), release of a tight thumb web, and so on may be necessary. If so, the appropriate aftercare is followed as described in the chapters pertaining to these conditions.

References and further reading

Carter, P. R. (1984) Crush injury of the upper limb: early and late management. *Orthopaedic Clinics of North America*, **14**, 719–747

Conolly, W. B., Morrin, J. and Davey, V. (1984) Mutilating injuries – postoperative care. In *Mutilating Injuries of the Hand*, 2nd edn (eds D. A. Campbell Reid, and R. Tubiana) Churchill Livingstone, Edinburgh, pp. 15–26

Davey, V., Conolly, W. B. and Masman, A. (1976) Clinical evaluation of the Masman pressure unit in the reduction of limb oedema. *Australian Journal of Physiotherapy*, **22**, 157–160

Green, D. P. (ed.) (1988) Microvascular surgery. In *Operative Hand Surgery*, vol. 2, 2nd edn (ed. D. Green) Churchill Livingstone, New York, pp. 1049–1330

Hunter, J. M., Schneider, L. H., Mackin, E. J. *et al.* (eds.) (1990) Trauma. In *Rehabilitation of the Hand: Surgery and Therapy*, 3rd edn, C. V. Mosby, St. Louis, pp. 167–263

Salter, M. I. (1987) Traumatic injuries. In *Hand Injuries: A Therapeutic Approach.* Churchill Livingstone, Edinburgh, pp. 118–172

11

Burnt hand

The most common burns are those from heat. Other types include frictional, electrical, chemical and radiation burns.

Exposure burns occur when the hand is used to protect the face or the rest of the body.

Contact burns occur when the hand grasps a hot object.

Pathological classification

There are three pathological types of burn. These are based on the depth of injury (Figure 11.1).

Superficial burns

Superficial burns are caused by scalding, an electric flash or

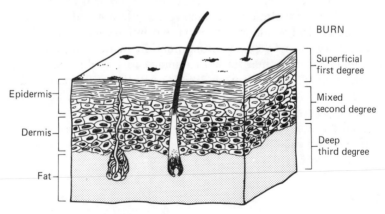

Figure 11.1 *Three depths of burn*

momentary contact with a radiator bar. They present with erythema (first degree) or blistering (second degree).

These burns are painful because the nerve endings remain uninjured. Deep epithelial cells survive and spontaneous healing occurs in 2–3 weeks, usually without the need for grafting.

Deep burns

Deep burns are caused by flames, friction, electricity or chemicals.

They destroy the epithelium and superficial nerve endings and are therefore painless. They have a greyish, waxy or charred appearance and heal by granulation tissue with scar formation. Skin grafting is usually necessary.

Mixed burns

Mixed burns can occur from any of the above causes.

In many burns there is a mixture of superficial and deep tissue damage.

Pathophysiology

The hand has a thin subcutaneous layer (i.e. poor insulation), thus facilitating heat conduction to important deeper structures. This is most marked on the dorsum of the hand and fingers where tendons and joints are close to the surface.

The hand also has a relatively large surface area and thus rapid heat gain in the dermal and subdermal layers can quickly overwhelm the microcirculation causing coagulation and thrombosis. Progressive ischaemia is added to the original thermal insult.

In every burn there is inflammation with congestion and oedema. Because there is both damage to the skin barrier and tissue damage, infection is likely. All these factors tend to predispose to fibrosis which may extend from the superficial layers to the muscles, tendons and joints, and even beyond the immediate area of the burn. It is not uncommon, therefore, for stiffness of a finger or the whole hand to occur even after a so-called minor burn.

Complications

1 Swelling.

2 Sepsis.
3 Ischaemia.
4 Scarring of skin, tendons or joints.
5 Contracture.

In the early postburn stage the main problem is sepsis or infection, which can convert a simple superficial burn to a dangerous deep one.

Most burns are surface-sterilized by the nature of the injury and thus those that become infected have been contaminated by the subsequent environment or by organisms in the glandular or follicular elements of the unburnt tissue. The burnt wound should be managed by the open method or by dressings to minimize the incidence of infection.

Later, stiffness becomes a problem. This is caused by inflammation, persistent oedema or poor positioning of the finger joints.

Other complications that may occur later on include mallet or buttonhole deformity from damage to the extensor apparatus over the DIP or PIP joints. Nail deformities can also be a problem.

Medical and nursing management of superficial burns

These burns are painful but they should heal spontaneously from epithelial remnants. The essentials of treatment are:

1 Control of pain with analgesia.
2 Prevention of infection by wound cleansing (Lux baths), with non-adherent and absorbent dressings, or by coating the burnt hand with an antibacterial cream and protecting it with a plastic bag. Systemic antibiotics are usually indicated as well as anti-tetanus cover.
3 Control of oedema by elevation of the hand.

Surgical management of deep burns

Because there are no epithelial remnants, healing occurs by granulation and scar tissue. The essentials of treatment are:

1 Surgical débridement of the burnt area.
2 Skin replacement by a graft or flap.

Surgical management of mixed burns

Here there is a mixture of epithelial regeneration and healing by scar. The essentials of treatment are:

(a)

(b)

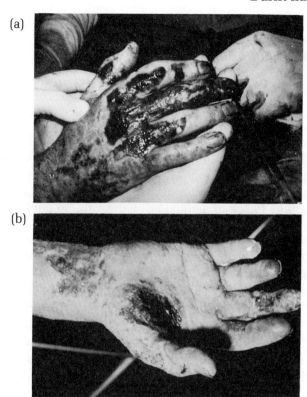

Figure 11.2   *(a) This 45-year-old publican suffered mixed burns to his right (dominant) hand while attempting to extinguish a hotel room fire. (b) Volar aspect showing deep (third degree) burn to the distal portion of the middle finger*

1 Initial treatment is as for superficial burns until the non-viable areas are demarcated.
2 The non-viable areas are excised and the defect is grafted (Figure 11.2a and b).
3 Hand is splinted in the POSI and elevated until the graft is stable (7–10 days).

Later reconstructive surgery

1 Scar revision by Z-plasty, grafting or a flap.
2 Nailbed reconstruction or ablation.

3 Extensor tendon repair or reconstruction for mallet or button-hole deformity.
4 Joint surgery for contracture. Capsulotomy or fusion in a functional position.
5 Amputation if there is irreparable damage to a digit.

Aims of therapy

1 Prevention of deformity.
2 Maintenance of joint movement.
3 Maintenance of mobility and use of all unaffected joints.
4 Restoration of maximum function.

Treatment measures for superficial burns

The hand is covered with an antibacterial cream such as silver sulphadiazine and protected by a plastic bag during the day (Figure 11.3). Light dressings are applied at night. This technique allows the patient to exercise and use the hand during the day for light selfcare activities, and minimizes the risk of stiffness.

Superficial burns are painful and analgesia before treatment is advisable.

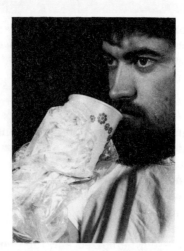

Figure 11.3 *Burnt hand is coated with silver sulphadiazine cream and covered with a plastic bag taped at the forearm. This enables the patient to carry out selfcare activity*

The hand is given three warm Lux baths daily. The therapist wears sterile rubber gloves and helps the patient perform the following exercises:

1 Wrist flexion and extension, and radial and ulnar deviation.
2 MCP joint flexion and extension.
3 Stabilized PIP and DIP joint flexion and extension followed by gross flexion and extension.
4 Finger abduction and adduction.
5 Opposition of the thumb to the pulp of each finger.

All exercises are performed very gently and slowly to avoid pain and soft tissue reaction.

The cream is washed off in the Lux bath. The hand is thoroughly rinsed in fresh warm water and then dried with sterile towels. The cream and plastic bag are then re-applied and the hand is splinted.

Early postburn splinting is vital to prevent the hand assuming the typical burnt-hand position of:

1 Wrist in flexion.
2 MCP joints in extension.
3 PIP joints in flexion, DIP joints in flexion or extension.
4 Thumb in adduction with IP joint in extension.

The hand is splinted as closely as possible in the POSI, i.e:

1 Wrist in 30–40 degrees extension.
2 MCP joints in maximum flexion.
3 IP joints in maximum extension.
4 Thumb in palmar abduction.

This splint is worn at night and during periods of inactivity throughout the day.

The initial splint may require frequent adjustment in response to oedema reduction.

Oedema is significant in most burns and the hand is therefore elevated at all times when not being exercised or used.

To encourage early functional use, adaptations of everyday utensils may be necessary, e.g. building up cutlery, razor and toothbrush handles.

Once the skin has epithelialized and there are no open areas, the cream and bag method is discarded.

The new skin is very fragile. It does not have any sebaceous secretion and is therefore dry and tends to crack easily. Lanolin or oil is smoothed gently into the skin to lubricate it. In the initial stages the skin must be protected from injury caused by friction, heat or ultraviolet rays.

On wound healing, the exercise programme is stepped up by giving resistance, which is gradually increased until maximum power has been regained.

A graded activity programme involving desensitization is implemented once resisted exercises are commenced.

An important part of the therapist's relationship with the patient involves emotional and psychological support.

Treatment measures for deep and/or mixed burns

Deep and/or mixed burns usually require excision of devitalized tissue followed by grafting (Figure 11.4).

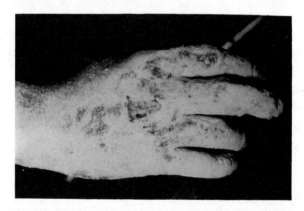

Figure 11.4   *Healing at 3 weeks following wound débridement and split skin grafting*

To prevent contractures during the time necessary for the graft to stabilize (that is about 1 week) the hand is immobilized as close to the POSI as the graft allows.

A deformity specific to deep dorsal burns is boutonnière (buttonhole) deformity, which is the result of damage to the extensor mechanism.

Care must be taken not to place undue tension on the finger extensor mechanism, and passive flexion is contraindicated when performing exercises (see below).

On graft healing, gentle active exercises are started. Initially these are performed in a warm Lux bath; this cleanses the wound and the warmth has the effect of reducing pain and facilitating movement. The following active exercises are begun:

1 Wrist flexion and extension, and radial and ulnar deviation.
2 MCP flexion and extension.
3 Finger abduction and adduction.
4 Stabilized PIP and DIP flexion and extension.
5 Thumb abduction, adduction, flexion and extension, and opposition to all digits.

All exercises are carried out within painfree limits. As pain decreases, and where there is no extensor tendon involvement, gross flexion exercises can be accompanied by gentle overpressure into flexion.

Later, graded resistance and passive stretching are added to the programme.

If there is extensor tendon damage, active exercises are carried out as follows, to prevent stretching or tearing of the extensor mechanism.

1 Maintenance of IP joint extension during MCP flexion.
2 Maintenance of MCP and DIP extension during PIP flexion.
3 Maintenance of MCP and PIP extension during DIP flexion.

The same technique applies to the thumb.

In between exercise sessions, IP extension can be maintained by means of volar or dorsal finger extension splints.

Where there is a tendency to thumb web tightness, gentle passive thumb web stretching is performed. Gains are maintained with foam wedges.

As healing progresses, there is a tendency to soft tissue tightness which may result in contractures. These are managed as follows:

1 For MCP extension contracture, an MCP flexion splint is used (Figure 11.5).
2 For PIP flexion contracture greater than 30–35 degrees an outrigger is used.
3 For an established thumb web contracture, a thumb outrigger can be incorporated into an MCP flexion splint (Figure 11.5) or dorsal outrigger, or serial C-splints may be used.

Healed raised scar tissue and/or persistent oedema are treated

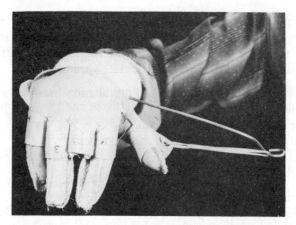

Figure 11.5 *Dorsal oedema and raised scar are treated with a Lycra pressure garment. Full digital MCP flexion and thumb extension are regained by the use of an MCP flexion splint incorporating a thumb outrigger*

with a Lycra pressure glove. Splints can be applied over the garment (Figure 11.5).

Both the glove and the splintage regimens may need to be maintained for up to 12–18 months, until the scar tissue becomes mature and no longer changes, and until joint mobility and tissue softness do not regress. Progress is assessed by gradual reduction in wearing time and evaluation of the response (Figure 11.6).

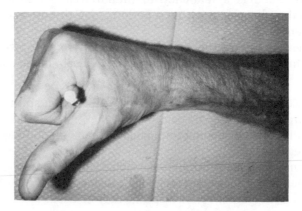

Figure 11.6 *Functional and cosmetic result at 8 weeks*

References and further reading

Blair, K. L. (1977) Prevention and control of hypertrophic scarring by the application of the custom-made Jobst pressure covers. *Jobst Institute*, Toledo, Ohio

Boswick, J. (1977) Burns and cold injury. In *The Hand: Surgical and Non-surgical Management* (eds E. S. Kilgore and W. P. Graham) Lea and Febiger, Philadelphia

Davis, A. T. (1987) The burnt hand. In *Hand Injuries: A Therapeutic Approach* (ed. M. I. Salter) Churchill Livingstone, Edinburgh, pp. 173–188

Fleegler, E. J. and Yetman, R. J. (1983) Rehabilitation after upper extremity burns. *Orthopaedic Clinics of North America*, **14**, 699–718

Hunter, J. M., Schneider, L. H., Mackin, E. J. *et al.* (eds.) (1990) Burns and cold injuries. In *Rehabilitation of the Hand: Surgery and Therapy*, 3rd edn, C. V. Mosby, St. Louis, pp. 831–864

Larson, D., Abston, S. and Evans, E. B. (1971) Splints and traction. In *Contemporary Burn Management* (eds H. Polk and H. H. Stone) Little, Brown, Boston

Malick, M. H. and Carr, J. A. (1982) *Manual on the Management of the Burn Patient*, Harmarville Rehabilitation Centre, Pittsburgh

12

Rheumatoid hand

Rheumatoid disease is the most common of the connective tissue disorders. It is really an inflammatory synovitis rather than an arthritis. By mechanical stretching and enzyme digestion, the synovitis:

1 Disrupts joint ligaments.
2 Erodes cartilage and subchondral bone.
3 Invades tendon mechanisms, restricting tendon glide and leading possibly to rupture.
4 When present in closed compartments, such as the carpal tunnel, causes secondary nerve compression.

These factors combine to cause pain, deformity and stiffness.

Rheumatoid disease can also be associated with skin nodules, purpura, vasculitis and intrinsic muscle fibrosis.

The disease is characterized by exacerbations and remissions.

Phases of rheumatoid disease

This condition, although it is a chronic systemic disease, can be arbitrarily divided into three clinical phases:

1 Inflammatory synovitis of joint and tendon mechanisms leading to pain, swelling and increased temperature (Figure 12.1).
2 Joint deformity with subluxation and/or dislocation, and intrinsic fibrosis (Figure 12.2).
3 Final remission (burnt-out rheumatoid disease). The degree of deformity and functional limitation varies from person to person (Figure 12.3).

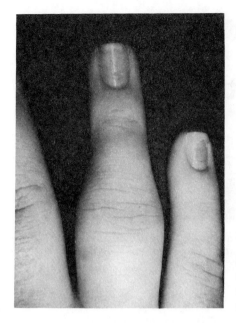

Figure 12.1 *Early rheumatoid arthritis is often characterized by fusiform swelling of the PIP joints*

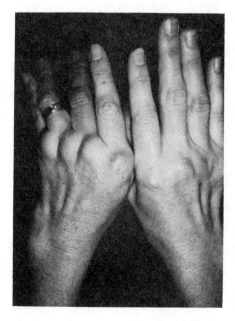

Figure 12.2 *Rheumatoid arthritis of the MCP joints (more severe in the left hand) with proliferative synovitis, ulnar deviation and MCP dislocation*

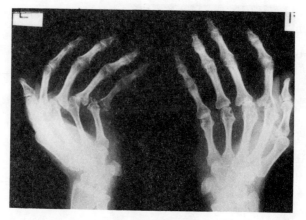

Figure 12.3 *Radiographic features showing diminished joint spaces, absorption of bone beneath the cortex adjacent to the joint, ulnar deviation of the fingers and MCP dislocation in the left hand*

Types of deformity

Metacarpophalangeal joints

Ulnar deviation (drift)

This occurs with or without volar subluxation and/or dislocation (Figure 12.3).

The tissues surrounding the joint, particularly the radial collateral ligaments, become permanently stretched as synovium proliferates and pushes against them.

The radial collateral ligaments are further damaged by the pull of the flexor tendons on the mouths of the flexor tendon sheaths in an ulnar direction. This ulnar pull by the flexor tendons causes dynamic ulnar drift.

The ulnar intrinsic muscles gradually become shortened, thereby increasing the pull toward ulnar drift.

MCP volar and ulnar subluxation results from synovitis stretching the extensor mechanism and causing the tendons to slip ulnarly and below the joint axes, thus acting as flexors rather than extensors.

Treatment

This depends on the degree of pain and/or functional disability (severe ulnar drift and subluxation are often compatible with excellent hand function in the absence of pain):

1 Synovectomy
2 MCP joint arthroplasty (replacement)

Proximal interphalangeal joint

Swan-neck deformity

This is hyperextension of the PIP joint with secondary flexion deformity of the DIP joint (Figure 12.4a and b).

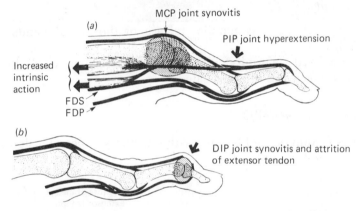

Figure 12.4 *(a) Swan-neck deformity in rheumatoid arthritis. MCP synovitis is associated with increased intrinsic muscle-tendon tension producing PIP hyperextension. (b) Swan-neck deformity and mallet deformity. Attrition of the extensor tendon from synovitis or trauma leads to mallet deformity*

Owing to flexor tendon synovitis the patient may experience difficulty flexing the PIP joint, resulting in the flexion effort being transmitted through the MCP joint instead. With the MCP joint in this flexed position the intrinsics are able to exert a greater pull through the central extensor tendon, thus creating an imbalance of hyperextension of the PIP joint.

In this position the volar plate is readily stretched, thereby increasing hyperextension. As this deformity develops, the lateral extensor tendons slip dorsally, further compounding the hyperextension problem.

The PIP deformity places the flexor digitorum profundus

tendon on the stretch resulting in a flexion deformity, which may be flexible or fixed, at the DIP joint.

The deformity is flexible if it is possible to flex the PIP joint with the MCP joint supported in extension. In this case there is only slight stretching of the volar plate.

The deformity is fixed (that is with tight intrinsic muscles) if PIP flexion can only be achieved with the MCP joint in the flexed position.

If full PIP flexion is not possible with the MCP joint flexed, the cause is adhesion of the extensor lateral bands.

Treatment

1 If the PIP joint is mobile, release of the lateral bands is indicated.
2 For a fixed deformity, PIP joint arthroplasty or fusion in a functional position is indicated.

Boutonnière deformity

This is flexion of the PIP joint with secondary hyperextension of the DIP joint (Figure 12.5).

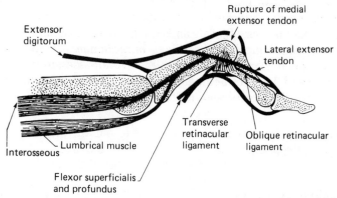

Figure 12.5 *Buttonhole deformity (rupture of the middle extensor tendon central slip of the extensor expansion). When this tendon is severed the PIP joint becomes flexed by the flexor superficialis and the subluxed lateral extensor tendons. These, with the oblique retinacular ligaments, hyperextend the DIP joint. Secondary contracture of the transverse retinacular ligaments and the volar plates causes a flexion contracture of the PIP joint*

Owing to proliferative synovitis of the PIP joint, the central extensor tendon is lengthened and weakened and may rupture, losing its extension effect on the PIP joint. The lateral bands fall below the axis of the joint, flexing rather than extending it. In this position the lateral bands are shortened, thus hyperextending the DIP joint.

Treatment

1 Early stage. PIP joint synovectomy, middle slip repair, and relocation of the lateral bands.
2 Later stage. PIP joint arthroplasty or fusion in a functional position.

Principles and types of management

Management of the rheumatoid patient requires a multidisciplinary approach involving the physician (rheumatologist), surgeon, therapists, orthotist and social worker.

Evaluation and treatment are an ongoing process because of the changing nature of the disease.

Involvement of hand structures cannot be viewed in isolation because the disabling effects of this disease are manifold, often involving a number of joints and other tissues or organs.

The psychological and social consequences of rheumatoid disease are vital considerations in the overall assessment.

Acute and long-term management of the rheumatoid patient can be broadly categorized under three headings.

1 Medical.
2 Therapeutic.
3 Surgical (see Surgery).

Medical management

Adequate rest forms part of the initial treatment. It can best be accomplished in the hospital environment where complete or partial bedrest can be enforced and physical activity can be limited to a degree in keeping with the local and systemic manifestations of the disease.

The drugs used to control rheumatoid synovitis include

salicylates, steroids, gold, antimalarials, cytotoxics and immuno-suppressants. Each may be effective in a particular patient but every drug has significant side-effects and the dosage must be carefully regulated.

Therapeutic management

The goals of therapeutic management are:

1 To maintain and/or increase joint mobility by gentle active and passive movements.
2 To maintain and/or increase muscle strength and endurance by isometric exercise and a carefully graded activity programme.
3 To prevent deformity by appropriate splintage and joint protection techniques.
4 To maintain and/or increase functional abilities by regular evaluation to determine the need for environmental modifications or the prescription of aids.
5 To educate the patient about his condition, i.e. to explain the treatment and the importance of maintaining mobility, and to give the reassurance that most people with this condition lead useful independent lives.

Gentle exercises are begun as soon as inflammation has subsided after bedrest and drugs.

Exercise periods are short and are carried out several times a day if possible. They include passive, active assisted and active movements, depending on patient tolerance.

Involved joints are splinted to provide rest and to maintain them in an anti-deformity position, e.g. splinting the knee in as much extension as possible or splinting the hand and wrist in the POSI (wrist in extension, MCP joints in flexion, IP joints in extension and thumb in palmar abduction; Figure 12.6).

Some patients benefit from the use of heat (wax baths) or cold (ice) treatment before exercise.

The patient is encouraged to participate in light non-resistive activity as soon as acute inflammation has subsided. Some rheumatologists prohibit any resistance beyond that necessary for selfcare, owing to the deforming forces of muscle contraction when joint structures are stretched and weakened. In keeping with this, pinch grip and power grip measurements and manual muscle testing should probably not be done.

A functional assessment is performed to examine all aspects of

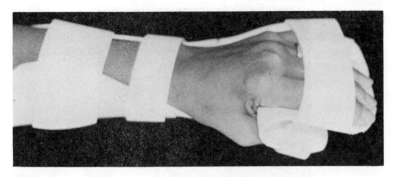

Figure 12.6   *During an exacerbation of rheumatoid disease the joints are protected by splinting the hand in the POSI*

the everyday needs of the patient to determine specific functional deficits. This assessment is repeated at regular intervals in accordance with changes in the condition.

Functional problems are managed by a combination of:

1 Aids and adaptations, and architectural modifications.
2 Splintage to enable optimum function.
3 Conservation of energy.
4 Work simplification.
5 Joint protection techniques.

Where possible, the assessment should be made in the patient's home or place of work. This gives a more realistic picture and allows planning of modifications.

Aids and adaptations

The initial evaluation involves an ADL assessment which examines the patient's ability to cope with selfcare activities such as feeding, bathing and toileting, dressing, personal grooming, getting in and out of bed, cooking and writing (Figure 12.7).

In prescribing aids and adaptations the aim is to restore maximum independence. For patient acceptance, aids should be well-designed, accurately fitted and as aesthetically pleasing as possible.

Some examples of aids and alterations are:

1 Enlargement of handles, e.g. cutlery, pen and key, and lengthening the handles of utensils such as comb and shoehorn.

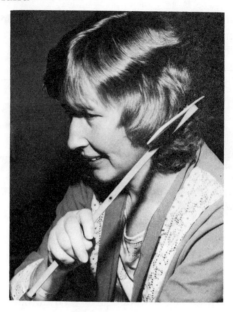

Figure 12.7   *Restriction of shoulder and elbow movements may necessitate the use of aids for grooming*

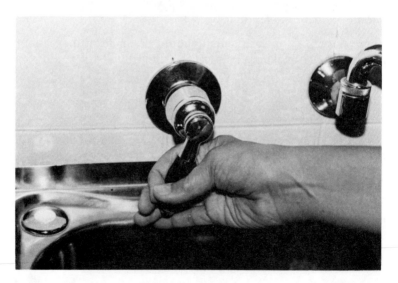

Figure 12.8   *Lever taps obviate the use of the small finger joints for tap turning*

2 Installation of lever-type taps and door handles, or use of a tap-turner (Figures 12.8 and 12.9).
3 Installation of handrails in bathroom/toilet.
4 Lightweight crockery and cooking utensils.
5 Spring-loaded scissors (Figure 12.10).
6 Raised toilet seat.

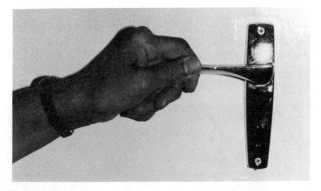

Figure 12.9 *Where possible door knobs should be replaced by lever handles for ease of grasp*

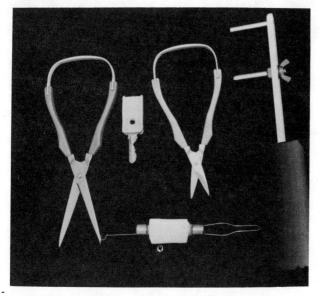

Figure 12.10 *Examples of aids including spring-loaded scissors, a built-up key, a padded buttonhook and a tap turner*

7 Velcro fastenings to replace buttons and zippers, or use of a buttonhook.
8 Raising of chair or bed to allow easy transfer.
9 Electrical labour-saving devices in the kitchen and laundry, such as a can-opener, knife and mixer.

Splintage

A painful and/or unstable wrist greatly inhibits hand function. A wrist cock-up splint provides pain relief and support while allowing maximum function (Figure 12.11).

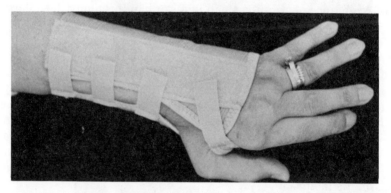

Figure 12.11   *Commercially available Pro-care elastic wrist brace is light and adjustable and provides firm wrist support during activity*

Conservation of energy and work simplification

As fatigue is a major symptom of rheumatoid disease, the daily and weekly home and work routine is planned so as to conserve energy and simplify work methods.

To avoid undue fatigue, a balance between rest and activity must be established. Where possible, use is made of extended and enlarged soft handles to decrease the grip force required to hold them. Major chores such as washing or cleaning are broken down into smaller manageable tasks. Whenever possible the patient sits to work. Commonly used foodstuffs and cooking utensils are stored in an accessible position.

Joint protection

The patient is taught to avoid deforming forces when using his hands in everyday activity.
Strain can be minimized by:

1 Avoidance of handling heavy objects, e.g. using a bookrest to hold a heavy book, and using a kitchen trolley to transfer items around the house.
2 Distributing a load over several joints at a time, e.g. lifting a teacup with two hands.
3 Using the strongest joint available for the task, for instance using a shoulder bag with a wide strap instead of a clutch purse, and carrying linen across the forearms.
4 Avoidance of gripping small items or handles tightly by enlarging their gripping surface, e.g. cutlery and key.
5 Avoiding any prolonged (static) grip that exerts force on a joint at one place, e.g. knitting.
6 Ensuring frequent rest periods during any activity.
7 Avoiding repeated jarring of joints, e.g. when using a heavy hammer.
8 Avoiding pressure that pushes the MCP or wrist joints in an ulnar direction, i.e. when stirring, both hands are used with a cylindrical grip and a circular motion of the entire arm rather than repeated ulnar deviation of the wrist; the chin is not rested on the hands.
9 Ceasing any activity that produces pain.

Surgery

General principles

The surgeon undertaking care of a patient with a rheumatoid hand problem must work in close liaison with a rheumatologist and with therapists experienced in this field.

In general, operative treatment is indicated if the patient has a particular disability and the surgeon can correct this without risk to existing function. The mere existence of deformity is not necessarily an indication for surgery: it is remarkable that a patient with rheumatoid disease can have advanced deformity and architectural disorganization of many joints and still have efficient hand function. Surgery can worsen the patient's hand function.

The deformed hand often retains good MCP joint flexion even in the presence of severe subluxation and ulnar drift at these joints.

The surgical programme is tailored to the individual patient. A careful assessment is fundamental. The surgeon-patient-therapist relationship is vital for a successful outcome.

Most rheumatoid patients have other joints and systems involved, and may require various surgical procedures.

Indications for surgical treatment

Pain relief

Synovectomy of joints or tendons is performed for persistent proliferative synovitis (Figure 12.12).

Restoration of function

This can be achieved by:

1 Repair or transplantation of ruptured tendons.
2 Arthrodesis or arthroplasty for joint disability.

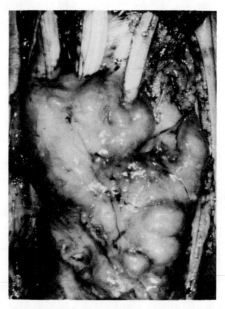

Figure 12.2 *Intraoperative photograph showing the rheumatoid proliferative pannus involving the extensor tendons*

Surgical priorities in the rheumatoid hand

Rheumatoid arthritis is a generalized disease often requiring an extensive surgical programme:

1 Extensor tenosynovectomy, excision of the ulnar head, and wrist stabilization.
2 Flexor tenosynovectomy.
3 MCP joint surgery.
4 PIP joint surgery and correction of finger deformities, e.g. swan-neck and boutonnière deformities.
5 Re-alignment of the thumb in the most useful position relative to the reconstructed fingers.

Surgical procedures

Joint synovectomy

Indications

Persistent painful synovitis unresponsive to medical treatment. The operation may prevent joint damage.

Technique

This procedure requires radical exposure of the joint so that all synovium from every area of the synovial cavity (not only the articular aspects) can be curetted.

Aftercare

Postoperative oedema is treated and, once this has subsided, early gentle exercises initially to maintain and then to increase the range of movement are begun.

Tenosynovectomy

Indications

Persistent painful tenosynovitis, flexor or extensor, with impaired tendon glide and the risk of tendon rupture.

Technique

The synovium from both outside and within the tendon is extensively resected while care is taken to preserve sufficient of the pulley system for mechanical leverage. (The involved tendons have an impaired blood supply, with subsequent risk of rupture.)

Aftercare

Early exercises are begun to prevent constrictive adhesions. These must be performed very gently to avoid rupture.

Tendon transplantation, repair or graft

Indications

Rupture of the extensor tendons to the ring or little fingers (Vaughan-Jackson syndrome) or to the thumb.

Technique and aftercare

The principles are the same as for other tendon surgery, but here there is a relatively poor blood supply and delayed healing of the repair. The exercise programme is, therefore, carried out very gently and slowly.

Silastic arthroplasty

See Chapter 7.

Ulnar head excision

Indications

Persistent painful dislocation of the ulnar head with or without extensor tendon rupture.

Technique

The distal end (2 cm) of the ulna is excised while preserving the overlying retinaculum, the extensor tendons and the fascial tissues. The ulnar head is replaced by a Silastic spacer and the overlying soft tissues are reconstructed.

Aftercare

To avoid dislocation, radioulnar rotation is prevented until the implant is encapsulated and the soft tissues are healed, i.e. for about 6 weeks.

Joint arthrodesis

Indications

Joint arthrodesis is used to stabilize a dislocated or extremely painful joint as an alternative to arthroplasty.

Technique

Because of poor bone stock (there is a significant incidence of non-union), standard arthrodesis procedures are modified by the addition of a bone graft, a compression technique or the use of a Harrison peg.

Aftercare

Prolonged immobilization is required and this is achieved by external or internal splintage. Mobility of the joints proximal and distal to the fused joint is maintained.

Intrinsic release

Indications

Tight intrinsic muscles across the PIP joint (swan-neck deformity) with an otherwise normal PIP joint mechanism.

Technique

Through a dorsal approach, each intrinsic expansion is dissected and either one or both expansions across the side of the proximal phalanx are incised sufficiently to enable full passive flexion of the PIP joint. (The tendon release is followed by fibrosis and a tendency to recurrence of intrinsic tightness.)

Aftercare

The corrected position is maintained by splintage, and early active exercises are commenced to prevent fibrosis and recurrence. (Wound healing following any surgical procedure may be impaired owing to the side-effects of prescribed drugs, e.g. corticosteroids, or to vasculitis and poor tissue nutrition.)

References and further reading

Brattstrom, M. (1973) *Principles of Joint Protection in Chronic Rheumatoid Diseases*, Wolfe, London

Ehrlich, G. E. (ed.) (1973) *Total Management of the Arthritic Patient*, J. B. Lipincott, Philadelphia

Flatt, A. E. (1974) *The Care of the Rheumatoid Hand*, 3rd edn, C. V. Mosby, St. Louis

Hunter, J. M., Schneider, L. H., Mackin, E. J. *et al.* (eds). (1990) Arthritis. In *Rehabilitation of the Hand: Surgery and Therapy*, 3rd edn, C. V. Mosby, St. Louis, pp. 885–949

Melvin, J. L. (1982) *Rheumatoid Disease, Occupational Therapy and Rehabilitation*, 2nd edn, F. A. Davis, Philadelphia

Nalebuff, E. A., Feldon, P. G. and Millender, L. H. (1988) Rheumatoid arthritis in the hand and wrist. In *Operative Hand Surgery*, vol. 3, 2nd edn (ed. D. P. Green) Churchill Livingstone, New York, pp. 1655–1764

Smith, R. J. and Kaplan, E. B. (1967) Rheumatoid deformities at the metacarpophalangeal joints of the fingers. *Journal of Bone and Joint Surgery*, **56A**, 85–91

Wynn Parry, C. B. (1981) The rheumatoid hand. In *Rehabilitation of the Hand*, Butterworths, London, pp. 355–376

13

Osteoarthritic hand

Osteoarthritis is the commonest arthritis to affect the hand. It most commonly affects the proximal and distal interphalangeal joints of the fingers and the carpometacarpal joint of the thumb.

Osteoarthritis is probably hereditary. This arthritis is commonest in post-menopausal women.

It can be primary in origin or secondary to a fracture or joint injury, e.g. post-traumatic osteoarthritis following a Bennett's fracture at the base of the first metacarpal.

Pathology

Osteoarthritis is not simply a failure of articular cartilage. It is a process which may involve all structures of the joint including subchondral bone, the synovium, the supporting ligaments and the neurovascular apparatus.

In the early stages, spurs develop along the joint margin and there is associated synovitis. At this stage, the cartilage can look reasonably healthy but histologically there is an active, synthetic mitotic process occurring in the cartilage.

Osteoarthritis is thus a biologically-mediated phenomenon and not just a wear-and-tear process. Arthritic tissue is biologically very active.

If a joint is immobilized for 6–8 weeks, the thickness of the cartilage is reduced and proteoglycans, the molecules that provide cartilage elasticity, are lost, with the bone becoming osteoporotic.

The cartilage no longer synthesizes the extracellular matrix responsible for the biomechanical functions of cartilage, such as the provision of smooth bearing surfaces and load transmission.

If the joint is then mobilized, the cartilage can return to normal within 3 weeks. In other words, cartilage actually heals.

Signs and symptoms

The signs and symptoms of osteoarthritis are the gradual onset of:

1 Pain.
2 Swelling.
3 Stiffness.
4 Instability.
5 Deformity.
6 Crepitation.
7 Weakness

Radiological changes do not necessarily correlate with the clinical picture; marked radiological changes can be seen in a patient with relatively few symptoms.

Occasionally, an acute and severe erosive osteoarthritis will present; the symptoms of pain, stiffness and deformity will be considerable in this case.

The characteristic bony outgrowths (osteophytes), which become prominent as the cartilage degenerates, are known as Bouchard's nodes at the PIP joint and Heberden's nodes at the distal IP joint (Figure 13.1).

General principles of treatment

Treatment aims to alleviate pain, improve the range of movement and increase functional ability.

Treatment can involve one or more of the following:

1 Hand therapy.
2 Drug therapy: anti-inflammatory agents, corticosteroid injections.
3 Surgery: arthrodesis, silastic implant arthroplasty, soft tissue
   arthroplasty.

Hand therapy

The acutely painful joint(s) can be splinted for a few days until symptoms subside.

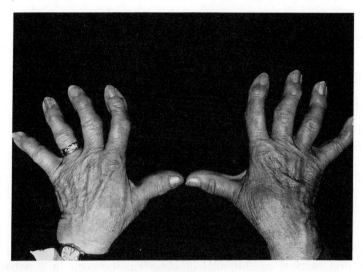

Figure 13.1 *Heberden's (DIP joint) nodes and Bouchard's (PIP joint) nodes are very evident in these osteoarthritic hands*

A POSI splint for night use and intermittent day wear provides comfortable support.

Heat, by way of warm water, heat packs or wax, can be an effective means of relieving pain and facilitating movement of stiffened joints.

Active exercises should be performed very gently and slowly and should not exacerbate pain. It is important to maintain the mobility of all upper limb joints. Passive exercise to the individual joints of the hand is not recommended as these tend to aggravate symptoms.

Gentle bandaging of the fingers into flexion using a wide, soft crepe bandage will assist in mobilizing the joints before active exercises. This position is maintained for approximately 20 minutes and the procedure can be repeated four to six times daily (Figure 13.2).

If the fingers are oedematous and painful, a Lycra pressure glove is often helpful in alleviating these symptoms (Figure 13.3).

For pain at the trapeziometacarpal joint (i.e. the first CMC joint), a thermoplastic thumb post can be worn at night (Figure 13.4).

When using the thumb, a soft neoprene splint is very effective

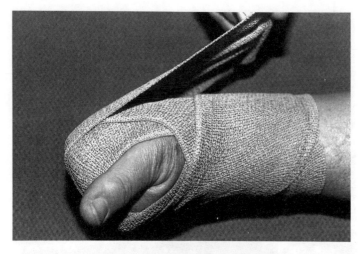

Figure 13.2 *Gently bandaging the fingers into flexion with a wide bandage before active exercise, assists in mobilizing the joints. Note that the wrist is held extended to facilitate finger flexion*

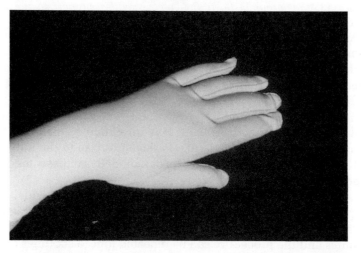

Figure 13.3 *Lycra pressure glove is worn to reduce oedema and provide some pain relief*

in providing support for this joint and thereby relieving pain. Some patients choose to wear the neoprene splint at night as well as during the day (Figure 13.5).

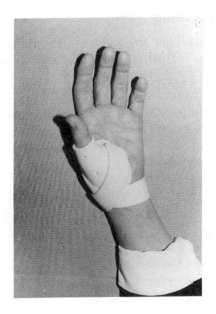

Figure 13.4 *Thermoplastic thumb post provides support to the first CMC joint*

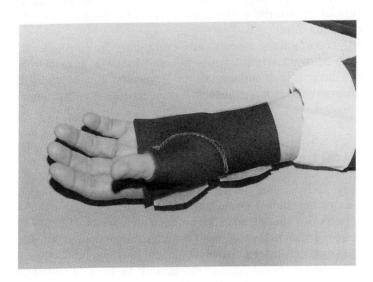

Figure 13.5 *Soft neoprene splint provides good support and pain relief and can be worn non-intrusively during activity*

Activities of daily living

Osteoarthritis involving the joints of the hand can seriously compromise hand function and often affects both pinch and power grip strengths.

Common complaints made by patients are:

1 Difficulty in placing a key in a lock and then turning it.
2 Difficulty with simple food preparation, e.g. the peeling of vegetables.
3 Inability to open jars and tins.
4 Inability to grasp cutlery.
5 Recreationally, inability to control a golf club or other sporting equipment.

Simple measures, e.g. the building-up of handles and the use of electric can openers, help to alleviate some of these problems. The building-up of keys with thermoplastic material overcomes the difficulty of unlocking doors.

Drug therapy

Pain in the joint produces inhibition of muscle power; therefore, the aim of pain relief with medication is to restore some of the power to the hand.

Anti-inflammatory agents are commonly prescribed. Local anaesthetic and corticosteroids injected into the joint give good relief from pain and inflammation. This relief may be short-lived but in many cases has significant duration. These injections can be repeated.

Surgical treatment

Surgery is indicated when functional and night pain are not satisfactorily relieved by the above measures.

Patients for surgery should be carefully selected. They must understand the nature of their problem and should appreciate what the procedure will involve.

It should be pointed out to the patient that while surgery will most likely improve function, it will not restore the hand to normal.

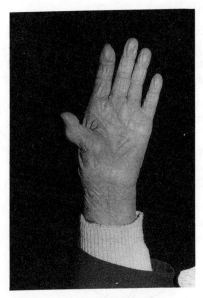

Figure 13.6 *Contracture of the first web space with secondary hyperextension of the MCP joint*

The most common surgical procedures are to the:

Carpometacarpal joint of the thumb

Osteoarthritis of this joint can result in painful instability of the thumb and a first web contracture; this often leads to secondary hyperextension of the MCP joint (Figure 13.6).
Surgical options include:

1 Implant arthroplasty which requires excision of the trapezium and its replacement by a silicone prosthesis or soft tissue implant (Figure 13.7).
2 If the arthritis is localized to the CMC joint, it can be fused.

NB If there is pantrapezial arthritis, i.e. involvement of the scaphotrapezial joint as well as the trapeziometacarpal joint, arthroplasty or fusion of this joint will not alleviate the problem.
The postoperative management of trapezium implant arthroplasty involves immobilization of the thumb and wrist in a thumb post for a period of 6 weeks; full thumb IP joint movement is allowed.

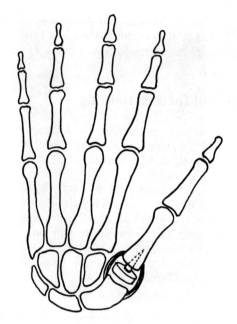

Figure 13.7   *Implant arthroplasty of the trapezium*

On removal of the splint, gentle active CMC joint movements are commenced.

Light non-resisted functional activity can be started, and approximately 3 months after operation the hand should be able to be used normally.

DIP joint

1 Fusion in a functional degree of flexion.
2 Occasionally, resection of osteophytes and bone spurs.

NB The DIP joint can stiffen spontaneously and will require no treatment if it is asymptomatic.

PIP joint

1 Very occasionally, PIP joint silastic implant arthroplasty to a single digit is indicated.

2 If there is pain and severe loss of flexion, and the patient rejects the idea of joint replacement, fusion in a functional position is an alternative, particularly for the index and little fingers.

References and further reading

Leonard, J. (1990) Joint protection for inflammatory disorders. In *Rehabilitation of the Hand: Surgery and Therapy*, 3rd edn (eds J. M. Hunter, L. H. Schneider, E. J. Mackin, *et al*). C. V. Mosby, St. Louis, pp. 908–911

Peimer, C. A. (1986) Osteoarthritis of the hand. In *Methods and Concepts in Hand Surgery* (eds N. Watson and R. J. Smith), Butterworths, London

Swanson, A. B. (1990) Pathogenesis of arthritic lesions. In *Rehabilitation of the Hand: Surgery and Therapy*, 3rd edn (eds J. M. Hunter, L. H. Schneider, E. J. Mackin, *et al*). C. V. Mosby, St. Louis, pp. 885–890

Swanson, A. B. and de Groot Swanson, G. (1983) Osteoarthritis in the hand. *Journal of Hand Surgery*, **8** (Part 2), 669

14

Reflex sympathetic dystrophy

Reflex sympathetic dystrophy (RSD), as defined by Lee Lankford, is a diseased state of an extremity that is characterized by:

1 Severe pain.
2 Swelling.
3 Stiffness.
4 Discoloration.

It usually occurs after trauma, surgery or disease and results from an abnormal sympathetic reflex or response.

Whilst this condition occurs infrequently, its early recognition and prompt and diligent treatment are vital if hand function is to be preserved.

RSD may be classified as:

1 Causalgia: with specific nerve injury.
2 Traumatic dystrophy: without specific nerve injury.
3 Shoulder-hand syndrome.

Causalgia

1 Major causalgia: involves injury to major nerves with resultant severe symptoms.
2 Minor causalgia: involves injury to a peripheral digital nerve and produces less severe symptoms and dysfunction.

Traumatic dystrophy

1 Major traumatic dystrophy: involves injury to soft tissue, joint

or bone without specific injury to any nerve; however, with severe symptoms of pain swelling, stiffness and discoloration.

2 Minor traumatic dystrophy: caused by injury to soft tissue, joint or bone with the resultant symptoms being less severe and possibly involving only a small segment of the hand.

Shoulder-hand syndrome

Shoulder-hand syndrome can follow trauma to the proximal part of the body or disease of, or damage to, a viscus, e.g. myocardial infarct.

RSD may be a consequence of any of the following:

1 Sprains.
2 Fractures.
3 Lacerations.
4 Crush injuries.
5 Amputations.
6 Burns.
7 Surgery (e.g. carpal tunnel decompression or fasciectomy for Dupuytren's contracture).

Wrist fractures are commonly associated with the onset of RSD owing to damage to the median nerve which carries most of the sympathetic nerve fibres to the hand.

There is considerable controversy as to whether certain personality types may be more prone to the development of RSD because they are more anxious, depressed or dependent.

Whether this is the case or not, it is important that these patients be handled with sensitivity, understanding and patience. As soon as the diagnosis of RSD is made, it should be explained to the patient and his or her family that this condition is an exaggerated and abnormal response to injury and one over which the patient has no control.

The patient with RSD will require ongoing support and referral to a skilled counsellor may be necessary.

Signs and symptoms of RSD

1 Pain.
2 Oedema.
3 Stiffness.

4 Vasomotor and pseudomotor changes.
5 Osteoporosis.
6 Trophic changes.

Pain

The pain experienced by a patient with RSD is often described as 'burning' and is of a severity which is out of all proportion to the degree of injury and/or surgery.

The nature of the pain may alter as the disease progresses. The patient will then use terms such as 'pressure-like', searing or aching.

Pain is aggravated by passive or active movements and changes in temperature. The patient may also experience dysaesthesia and paraesthesia when light touch is applied to the affected skin. Pain affects the hand, wrist and forearm and is usually worse around the IP joints of the fingers.

Oedema

Oedema is at first soft and obliterates all joint creases. It involves the fingers, hand and distal forearm (Figure 14.1).

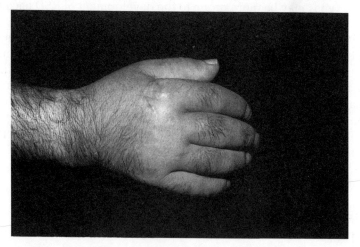

Figure 14.1 *Early stage of RSD showing soft, 'puffy' oedema which obliterates joint creases*

As time progresses the oedema becomes thickened and brawny and contributes significantly to loss of movement.

Stiffness

This is initially the inability to move the joints passively or actively because of the severity of the pain.

In later stages stiffness is the result of brawny oedema and subsequent fibrosis which impedes tendon glide and intrinsic muscle function. The fibrous structures around the joints lose their elasticity and become thickened and rigid.

Vasomotor and pseudomotor changes

The patient may present with a discoloured hand which is either red and warm (from vasodilation) or pale, cool and cyanotic (from vasoconstriction).

A reddened hand, particularly on the dorsum of the MCP and IP joints, appears to be the more common presentation.

Hyperhidrosis (excessive sweating) may be seen in the early stages and is often associated with a decrease in temperature.

Skin dryness is usual in the later stages of the disease. In some very severe cases of RSD, dryness may occur in the early stages with an associated increase in skin temperature.

Osteoporosis

In the early stages of the disease, osteoporosis is seen in the polar regions of the long bones, i.e. the metacarpals and the phalanges. In more severe cases of RSD, osteoporosis is evident in the carpal bones giving a spotted appearance which may progress to a picture of diffuse osteoporosis if the condition is left untreated.

Trophic changes

The skin of a patient with RSD is usually shiny. In the early stages this is caused by the oedema and smoothing out of the skin creases together with lack of joint movement.

In later stages, the glossy appearance results from nutritional changes caused by skin and subcutaneous tissue atrophy. The fat pads at the tips of the fingers atrophy causing the nails to curve downward giving a 'pencil-pointing' appearance. The nails become thickened, rigid and brittle and hair becomes coarse.

Clinical course of RSD

RSD may run through clinical stages.

Stage 1

In the early phase of stage 1, burning pain is the paramount symptom and continues throughout this stage, often increasing in severity.

Oedema is very noticeable and loss of movement is also apparent. Light touch often produces an exquisitely painful response (allodynia).

Vasomotor and pseudomotor changes usually produce a pale, cool or cyanotic hand with excessive sweating at this early stage. This later changes to red discoloration with dry skin and increased skin temperature.

Osteoporosis does not usually become evident until the fifth week. It has a spotty appearance with demineralization occurring in the polar regions of the metacarpals and phalanges and also in the carpal bones.

Stage 1 lasts for approximately 3 months.

Stage 2

Pain persists and increases in severity if left untreated. It is aggravated by active and/or passive movement.

Oedema changes from being soft to brawny and hard and is resistant to the usual methods of oedema control. Stiffness becomes more marked (Figure 14.2).

Vasomotor changes produce redness and increased temperature, and there is decreased sweating.

Osteoporosis changes from being spotty to becoming more diffuse.

The skin takes on a more glossy appearance.

This stage usually lasts up to 9 months.

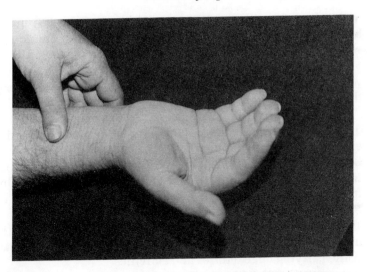

Figure 14.2 *Marked stiffness in stage 2 of RSD*

Stage 3

Pain remains a constant problem for several months but sometimes slowly decreases. If pain does still persist, it has usually reached its maximum severity at this stage.

Pain may continue for up to 2 years and sometimes continues indefinitely.

Oedema that was present in stage 2 changes to obvious thickening of all structures around joints (periarticular thickening).

The hand appears glossy and pale and feels dry and cool. There is obvious skin and subcutaneous atrophy.

Osteoporosis is very severe and the hand is rendered virtually useless.

Treatment

This may involve the use of:

1 Somatic nerve blocks: these are suitable for the minor types of RSD, i.e. minor causalgia and minor traumatic dystrophy. A local anaesthetic agent (Xylocaine, Marcaine) is administered at wrist level into the median, ulnar or radial nerve, or occasionally as an axillary block.

2 Stellate ganglion blocks: a successful block will result in the hand becoming warm and dry, with a return of more normal skin colour. There is usually also marked pain relief.

Stellate ganglion blocks are usually given once or twice a week and on average, four or five blocks are required to reverse the abnormal sympathetic reflex.

The relief derived from a successful block may last from 1 to 3 days and it is during this period that gentle passive and active exercises should be employed.

3 Regional intravenous sympathetic blockage: e.g. intravenous infusion of guanethidine. This acts by blocking noradrenaline from the sympathetic nerve terminals.

4 Sympatholytic drugs: e.g. reserpine, guanethidine.

5 Transcutaneous electrical nerve stimulation: TENS should be used over the trigger points and the patient can wear the device while carrying out exercises and activities.

6 Surgical sympathectomy.

Hand therapy

The appropriate therapy measures to overcome oedema and stiffness should be instituted as soon as pain relief has been achieved.

It must be noted that the use of passive exercises without previous pain relief will exacerbate the patient's symptoms and make the stiff, swollen joints even more stiff and painful.

Exercises practised by the patient should be performed on an hourly basis and should be carried out in a sustained and systematic fashion.

Active, stabilized interphalangeal flexion exercises with a strong 'pull-through' must be encouraged.

If at all possible, the wrist should be splinted into extension; not only is this position important for function, it also facilitates effective finger flexion (Figure 14.3).

Serial thermoplastic splinting can be gently employed to overcome wrist stiffness.

Where MCP joint extension contractures and/or PIP joint flexion contractures have developed, one must first achieve some wrist extension in order to overcome these contractures.

It is most important to remember that any splint used, be it static or dynamic, must not result in increased pain or swelling (Figure 14.4).

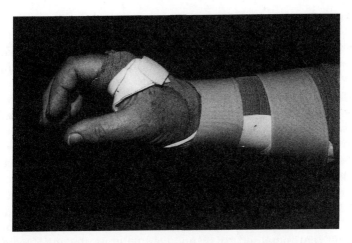

Figure 14.3 *The wrist should, if at all possible, be splinted in extension. This position is most important for function as well as facilitating effective finger flexion.*

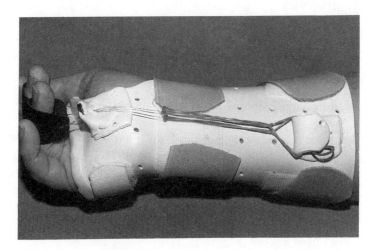

Figure 14.4 *Dynamic splints to correct joint contractures are often needed once the pain cycle has been brought under control*

Light, functional activity should be encouraged in conjunction with the exercise and splinting programme. Activities suggested should be realistic and easily achievable by the patient so as to encourage morale.

'Stress loading' programme

A non-invasive treatment programme, offering an alternative to the pharmacological/chemical or surgical approach, has been put forward by Kirk Watson.

The programme is based on active 'stress loading' which consists of active traction and compression exercises that provide stressful stimuli to the extremity without joint movement.

Kirk Watson has prescribed this programme alone for his RSD patients over the past 20 years and its advantages are that it is simple, safe and often effective.

Passive and active movements, or other therapy methods, are not implemented until pain and oedema have begun to subside.

At the commencement of the programme, it is explained to the patient that increased pain and swelling are to be anticipated in the first few days but that they should begin to decrease after this time.

Method

Scrub

The patient assumes the quadruped position on the floor with a coarse-bristled scrubbing brush held in the affected hand. With the patient leaning on the arm, he or she begins scrubbing a plywood board, applying as much pressure as possible and using a backward-forward motion.

Where it is impractical or difficult for the patient to assume the quadruped position, or if he or she is unable to achieve sufficient wrist extension to control a brush, scrubbing can be performed on a table top, or the brush be substituted with a polishing cloth.

The home programme involves 3 min of steady scrubbing or polishing, three times daily (Figure 14.5).

Carry

The patient carries a bag or purse in the affected hand while holding the arm in the extended position. If the patient has insufficient flexion to gain purchase on a bag handle, a plastic bag can be looped around the wrist in a figure-of-eight fashion.

The amount of weight used is determined by the maximum weight that the patient can tolerate. Initially, this is approximately 0.5 kg and is gradually increased to 2.25 kg in weight.

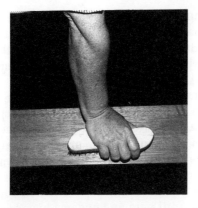

Figure 14.5 *'Scrubbing' component of the stress-loading programme*

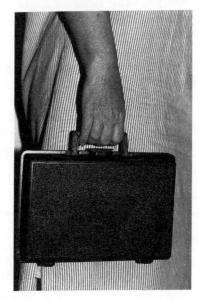

Figure 14.6 *'Carry' component of the stress-loading programme*

The weight is carried whenever the patient is walking or standing (Figure 14.6).

A daily record is kept of any weight increments and the patient's progress is monitored on a daily or second-daily basis during the first week.

Improvement in the hand is usually observed approximately 5 days after the commencement of treatment.

After several days, the 'scrub' component of the programme is increased to 5 minutes, three times daily. It is increased to 7-min sessions after approximately 2 weeks.

It is important to check that adequate pressure is being applied throughout the 'scrubbing' process and that the patient is able to tolerate the increase in session times.

It is only when the pain has subsided that other treatment methods such as gentle exercise and splinting are added to the programme.

Summary

In summary, reflex sympathetic dystrophy is generated by an abnormal sympathetic response which is at present still poorly understood.

RSD is an active disease process, the main features of which include pain, stiffness, swelling and discoloration, which are often out of all proportion to the antecedent injury or disease.

It is important to realize that not all painful, red, swollen and stiff hands are the result of RSD. The diagnosis can be confirmed by way of a stellate ganglion block which should relieve pain, warm the hand and return the skin to a more normal colour. Several of these blocks may be necessary before a definitive diagnosis is made.

Early diagnosis, referral and treatment are the keys to successful management of this condition. Rehabilitation of the patient usually requires multiple therapeutic interventions, including both invasive and non-invasive techniques.

Because of a patient's predisposition to this disease, any late-stage elective surgery, e.g. capsulotomies, should only be performed in conjunction with a precautionary stellate ganglion block or sympathectomy.

References and further reading

Glynn, C. J., Basedow, R. W. and Walsh, J. A. (1981) Pain relief following post-ganglionic sympathetic blockade with i.v. guanethidine. *British Journal of Anaesthesia*, **53**, 1297

Lankford, L. L. (1988) Reflex sympathetic dystrophy. In *Operative Hand Surgery*, vol. 1, 2nd edn (ed. D. P. Green) Churchill Livingstone, New York, p. 633

Lankford, L. L. (1990) Reflex sympathetic dystrophy. In *Rehabilitation of the Hand: Surgery and Therapy*, 3rd edn (eds J. M. Hunter, L. H. Schneider, E. J. Mackin *et al*). C. V. Mosby, St. Louis, pp. 763–786

Stanton-Hicks, M., Jänig, W. and Boas, R. A. (eds) (1990) *Reflex Sympathetic Dystrophy* (Current Management of Pain, P. Prithvi Raj, Series Editor), Kluwer Academic Publishers, Boston.

Watson, H. K. and Carlson, L. (1987) Treatment of reflex sympathetic dystrophy of the hand with an active 'stress loading programme.' *Journal of Hand Surgery*, **12A(5)** (part 1), 779

Waylett-Rendall, J. (1990) Therapist's management of reflex sympathetic dystrophy. In *Rehabilitation of the Hand: Surgery and Therapy*, 3rd edn (eds J. M. Hunter, L. H. Schneider, E. J. Mackin, *et al*). C. V. Mosby, St. Louis, pp. 787–792

15

Splinting in hand therapy

Baillière's Nurses' Dictionary defines a splint as: 'an appliance used to support or immobilize a part while healing takes place or to correct or prevent deformity'.
Splints may be either static or dynamic.

Static

A static splint has no moving components and provides support to a joint(s) in one position.
Static splints can be used in a dynamic way by applying the splint at the maximum range of joint movement; this position is then modified every few days. When this method is employed, it is termed serial static splinting.
Static splints are used for the following reasons:

1 Protection: e.g. a dorsal splint maintaining wrist and finger flexion following flexor tendon repair.
2 Immobilization: e.g. a thumb post following ligamentous damage to the MCP joint of the thumb.
3 Support: e.g. a POSI splint is used during the 'flare-up' period in rheumatoid disease; a neoprene thumb support for the osteoarthritic thumb.
4 Positioning: e.g. the crushed hand is placed as closely as possible in the POSI to prevent a 'claw' deformity resulting from dorsal hand oedema.
5 Correction: e.g. a C-splint used serially to stretch the first web space.
6 To gain optimum hand function: e.g. a simple wrist cock-up splint facilitates hand function for the 'wrist drop' hand in a

ıerve palsy; a thumb rotation strap opposes the thumb
:h grip function in a low-level median nerve lesion.

Dynamic

A dynamic splint achieves its effect by movement and force and
is a form of manipulation.

The splint may use forces which are applied externally as in
the case of rubber bands and coils, or those which are generated
by the patient's own muscles.

Dynamic splints can be used to:

1 Mobilize stiff joints: e.g. an MCP joint flexion splint to overcome an MCP joint extension contracture; a PIP joint outrigger
   extension splint to overcome a PIP joint flexion contracture.
2 Prevent contractures in nerve palsies by controlling deformity:
   e.g. a 'spaghetti' splint which reverses hyperextension of the
   MCP joints in an ulnar nerve 'claw' deformity.
3 Substitute for absent muscle power or to assist weak muscles:
   e.g. an outrigger splint for radial nerve palsy 'wrist-drop'.
4 Maintain alignment: following MCP joint arthroplasty.
5 Overcome soft tissue tightness and/or adhesions: e.g. an outrigger which stretches contracted muscle-tendon units following
   flexor tendon/nerve surgery at the wrist.

Classification

1 Forearm-based/hand-based/finger-based.
2 Volar/dorsal.
3 Rigid (i.e. thermoplastic or plaster of Paris)/soft (i.e. neoprene,
   Velfoam, leather).

Patient education

Patient compliance is fundamental to the success of any splinting
regimen. The patient must understand:

1 The purpose for which the splint has been prescribed.
2 Its correct application.
3 The need for regular review, particularly in the case of dynamic
   splints where outrigger modifications are made frequently.
4 The importance of checking the skin for pressure areas,

compromised circulation or swelling, and reporting these promptly to the therapist. This is especially important for patients with impaired sensation.

5 That a splint should not cause pain. In the case of a mobilizing splint, the patient should experience a stretching sensation which may be a little uncomfortable but is necessary for overcoming joint stiffness.

6 That dynamic splints should be worn intermittently; they should be removed at regular intervals throughout the day and all relevant joints should be put through their range of movement.

7 That splints, particularly dynamic ones, are an adjunct to, not a substitute for, hand therapy. Splints do not abolish the need for a structured exercise/activity programme.

To help ensure patient compliance, splints should where possible be:

1 Simple in design.
2 As comfortable as possible.
3 Lightweight.
4 Easy to put on and take off.
5 Free of pressure areas.
6 As cosmetically pleasing as possible.
7 Readily adjustable.

General principles for the making of forearm-based splints

1 The Splint should follow the contour of the hand and forearm and maintain the arches of the hand (Figure 15.1).

2 To ensure even distribution of pressure, the width of the forearm piece, either dorsal or volar, should extend as far as the lateral and medial midlines of the forearm; to ensure stability of the wrist and hand, the splint should extend to two-thirds of the length of the forearm.

3 The Length of the splint is determined by the joint(s) whose movement should be maintained, e.g. a wrist cock-up splint should finish proximal to the distal palmar flexion crease to permit full flexion of the MCP joints; unless there is thumb ray involvement, the CMC and MCP joints of the thumb should be allowed to move freely (Figure 15.2).

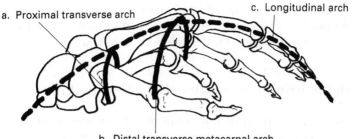

a. Proximal transverse arch

c. Longitudinal arch

b. Distal transverse metacarpal arch

Figure 15.1 *The arches of the hand: (a) proximal transverse arch; (b) distal transverse metacarpal arch; (c) longitudinal arch*

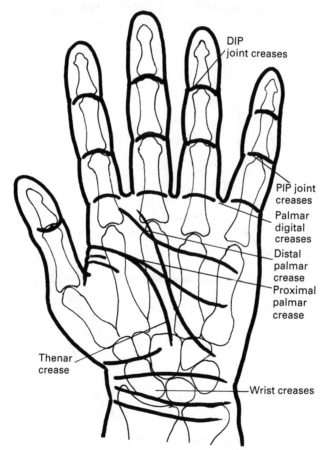

DIP joint creases

PIP joint creases

Palmar digital creases

Distal palmar crease

Proximal palmar crease

Thenar crease

Wrist creases

Figure 15.2 *Skin creases of the palmar aspect of the hand in relation to the underlying bones*

4 To prevent restriction of elbow movement and pressure on the cubital blood vessels, the proximal limit of the splint should be about four finger-widths below the elbow joint.

Specific principles of dynamic splint-making

1 The static portion of the splint should fit very well to avoid splint migration or rotation when forces are applied.
2 The bone proximal to the joint being mobilized should be well stabilized, e.g. the proximal phalanx must be stabilized when making an outrigger to overcome a PIP joint flexion contracture.
3 The line of pull should be at a right angle to the axis of the skeletal segment being moved (Figure 15.3).

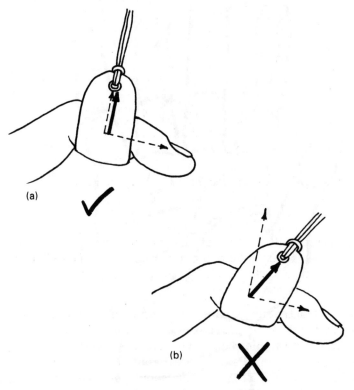

(a)

(b)

Figure 15.3   *When applying rubber band traction, the line of pull should be at a right angle to the axis of the skeletal segment being moved. (a) Correct. (b) Incorrect*

4 During flexion, the fingers converge toward the scaphoid bone (Figure 15.4). When applying a flexion force to a digit, ensure that the line of pull is in this direction.

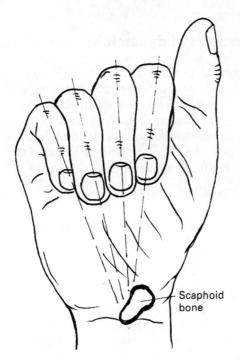

Figure 15.4 *During flexion the fingers converge towards the scaphoid bone*

5 When correcting joint or soft tissue contractures, the tension of the rubber bands should produce a force that is sufficient to effect change, yet sufficiently low so as not to incite an inflammatory reaction.

The tension of the rubber bands is determined by their length and thickness. Long, thin rubber bands will produce relatively low forces while short, thick bands will produce high forces.

For finger traction, Paul Brand (Brand, 1990) recommends a force in the vicinity of 200 g; this should be measured using a spring scale (Figure 15.5).

Because of their fatiguability, rubber bands should be replaced regularly.

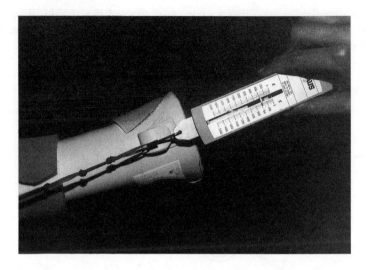

Figure 15.5 *Spring scale is used to measure force when applying rubber band traction*

The goal for the patient using a corrective dynamic splint is to tolerate the splint for increasing periods of time, not increasing degrees of force, i.e. to maintain a 'prolonged state of mild tension'. This is achieved by using rubber bands producing low forces.

Dynamic splints prescribed to overcome joint or soft tissue tightness are ideally worn throughout the night and on a 1 h-on/2 h-off basis throughout the day.

Initially, 3–6 h at night may be all that can be tolerated; this time is then gradually increased in accordance with the patient's tolerance of the splint.

NB Some indication of the potential for mobilizing a stiff joint can be gleaned by assessing the 'end-feel' of the joint.

If there is a 'springy' feel at the end of the joint's maximum passive range, then this is an encouraging sign. If, however, the joint can be moved to a certain point and then stops in a sudden, non-yielding manner, it is said to have a 'hard end-feel' and conservative treatment may be useless; even so, it is usually worth attempting a conservative approach for a number of weeks before surgery is embarked upon.

Equipment, tools and materials

Equipment

1 Heating pan (hydrocollator).
2 Heat gun.
3 Sewing machine (ideally a light industrial machine to cope with leather, Velcro and neoprene).
4 Shadow board for tools.

Tools

1 Stanley knife.
2 Splinting shears.
3 Scissors (suitable for cutting Velcro, leather, neoprene).
4 Leather punch.
5 Wire snips.
6 Plaster of Paris saw.
7 Jig for coil-making.
8 Long-nosed pliers.
9 Wire bender (for outrigger wires).
10 Tongs (padded so as not to mark the thermoplastic materials).

Materials

1 Paper towelling for patterns.
2 Towels for drying thermoplastic materials before their application.
3 Thermoplastic materials: San-Splint XR, Ezeform, Custom-splint, Orfit (these materials represent only a small selection of what is available).
4 Plaster of Paris.
5 Leather: should be very soft and flexible.
6 Neoprene (wet-suit material): for thumb supports or flexion straps.
7 Tubigrip stockinette (usually sizes A–F) for skin protection beneath the splint and oedema control.
8 Tubifast green stockinette.
9 Lycra: for fingerstall manufacture.
10 Velcro: hook and pile, 2.5 and 5 cm, adhesive and non-adhesive, elastic and non-elastic.
11 Velfoam: for strapping.

12 Lining foams: Luxofoam, Kushionflex, Polycushion.
13 Moleskin.
14 Spring-steel wire (17 Guage) for Capener splint.
15 Nylon fishing line: for low-profile splints.
16 Rubber bands of various sizes for traction.
17 Wire for outriggers (coat-hanger or copper wire).
18 Safety pins of various lengths: for pulleys when making low-profile flexion splints.
19 'Zoff' solvent (adhesive plaster remover): to clean surfaces of thermoplastic materials in preparation for bonding.

The thermoplastic splints described in this chapter have been made from San-Splint XR, Ezeform or Orfit (thinnest gauge).

As has been stated, these materials are representative of a large number of materials available on the market. They are low-temperature thermoplastic materials and the authors have found them to fulfil most of their splinting needs.

Care should be taken not to overheat the materials as they become too 'stretchy'. Softened materials for large splint patterns should be removed from the heating pan very carefully and in a horizontal fashion so that the material does not lengthen.

With the exception of Ezeform, these drapable materials should be allowed to almost 'fall' into the desired position with only the gentlest stroking actions being used to mould into place where necessary. Pressure from the tips of the fingers should be avoided as this will result in indentation of the material with resultant pressure areas.

Where more rigidity is required, e.g. when making serial C-splints or a volar pan splint to stretch tight structures, Ezeform is a more suitable material as it does not mark or indent easily when handled.

The drapability of these materials and the contiguous fit provided by them obviates the need for lining in most cases.

Areas of the splint to which adhesive Velcro hook is to be applied or where bonding of materials should occur, can be prepared with 'Zoff' solvent (adhesive plaster remover) and the area scored with a Stanley knife for better bonding.

Straps for securing splints should be of an appropriate width to ensure an even distribution of pressure and therefore comfort.

Because of the bony prominences at the wrist, straps at this level should be of Velfoam or well-padded Velcro pile.

Volar wrist cock-up (extension) splint.

See Figures 5.6 and 15.6.

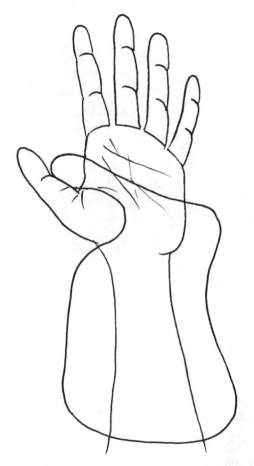

Figure 15.6 *Pattern for volar wrist (extension) cock-up splint*

Indications

1 To support a painful or weak wrist resulting from injury, rheumatoid disease or osteoarthritis.
2 As a serial splint for gradual correction of a flexion contracture of the wrist following tendon and/or nerve repair at wrist level.

3 To alleviate the symptoms of carpal tunnel syndrome, that is, compression of the median nerve at the wrist.
4 As the basis of a dynamic MCP joint flexion splint to correct MCP joint extension contractures (Figure 15.7).

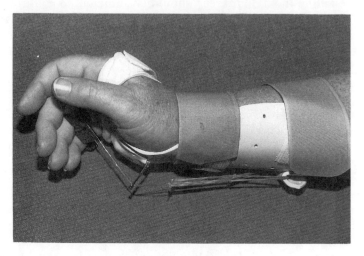

Figure 15.7   *Dynamic low-profile MCP joint flexion splint*

Low-profile MCP joint flexion splint

Materials

1 Soft leather for finger loops.
2 Nylon fishing line.
3 Safety pins for pulleys.
4 Rubber bands (thin) for traction.

Construction

When the line and angle of pull have been established, a safety pin of appropriate length is bent with long-nosed pliers; the 'sharp' end of the pin which is to be attached to the splint is heated over a heat gun while it is held in the pliers. It is then gently embedded in the splint and a small piece of thermoplastic material is bonded on to this area for both cosmesis and to prevent the pin from dislodging.

The width of the leather loops should extend from the inter-digital web space to the level of the PIP joint for even distribution of pressure.

Holes are punched at both ends of the leather loop and nylon fishing line is threaded through the ends, creating a 'parachute'. The length of the nylon thread should be sufficient to go through and reach just beyond the hole of the safety pin. The extra length beyond the safety pin is required for when the patient extends against the rubber bands so that there is sufficient excursion of the nylon thread in the pulley.

At this level, rubber bands are attached to the nylon thread; these are then attached to a hook which has been bonded on to the proximal end of the splint.

NB If more than one digit is involved, it may be necessary to use several safety pins of differing lengths to accommodate the varying lines and angles of pull for each digit.

For a PIP joint flexion splint, the outrigger pattern (Figure 15.9) can be used on the volar aspect of the hand with the splint finishing just proximal to the PIP joints to allow for their flexion.

The 'wing' portion at the distal end of the splint secures the MCP joints in extension to avoid them being flexed when the traction is applied to the middle phalanges.

Pan resting splint

See Figure 15.8.

Indications

1 Whenever rest and immobilization are indicated, e.g. in acute rheumatoid disease, stable fractures of the hand and soft tissue injury. This splint maintains the hand in the POSI, i.e. wrist in 30–40 degrees extension, MCP joints in maximum flexion, IP joints in maximum extension and the thumb (where necessary) in palmar abduction (see Figures 0.2 and 12.6).
2 This splint can be used as a volar stretch splint (Figure 9.7) to overcome flexor tightness or to maintain and/or improve extension following fasciectomy for Dupuytren's disease. The thumb piece is omitted and the wrist positioned in neutral. A wide Velfoam strap applies pressure over the dorsum of the PIP or MCP joints, depending on where the flexor tightness is more prevalent.

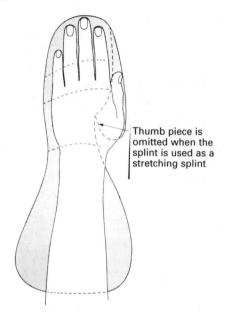

Thumb piece is
omitted when the
splint is used as a
stretching splint

Figure 15.8   *Pattern for pan resting splint*

Interphalangeal joint flexion strap

See Figure 5.9.

Indications

To achieve the last 15–30 degrees of IP joint flexion, particularly
of the DIP joint.

Materials

1 Strip of Velfoam measuring approximately 3 cm in width and
   16 cm in length.
2 Square of non-adhesive Velcro hook measuring 3 × 3 cm.

Construction

1 Velcro hook is sewn to one end of the velfoam strip.
2 The affected digit is gently flexed passively at both IP joints to

their maximum pain-free limit and the strap is drawn around the digit and attached to itself.

If there is insufficient flexion of the IP joints to apply a digit-based flexion strap, a hand-based flexion strap can be used until sufficient flexion range has been gained to enable use of the digit-based strap (see Figure 2.17). The length and width of this strap needs to be increased for the hand-based design.

Dorsal outrigger (low-profile design)

See Figure 15.9.

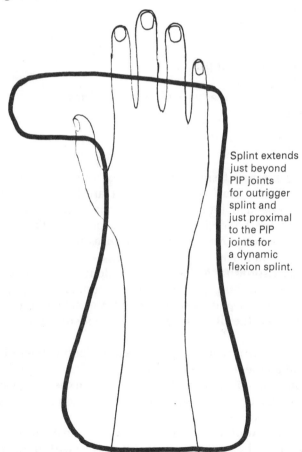

Splint extends just beyond PIP joints for outrigger splint and just proximal to the PIP joints for a dynamic flexion splint.

Figure 15.9 *Pattern for dorsal outrigger*

Indications

1 PIP joint flexion contracture greater than 45 degrees that is strongly resistant to passive extension.

Splint position:

 (a) Wrist in 35–45 degrees of extension.

 (b) MCP joints in maximum flexion.

2 Postoperative or postinjury soft tissue tightness in the distal palm leading to a flexion deformity of the MCP and PIP joints simultaneously.

Splint position:

 (a) Wrist in neutral.

 (b) MCP joints as close to neutral position as possible (see Figure 9.8).

Materials

1 Leather for finger loops.
2 Nylon fishing line.
3 Coat-hanger or copper wire for outrigger arms.
4 Rubber bands.

Construction

The outrigger arm is fashioned by hand or with a wire bender.

The proximal 'arms' of the outrigger are heated over a heat gun and embedded into the splinting material in the position appropriate to the digits involved. A piece of thermoplastic material is bonded over the exposed wires for cosmesis and to hold the wire in place.

A piece of splinting material is then double-bonded on to the distal frame of the outrigger. When the material has cooled, a hole is punched at that point where a 90-degree angle of pull will be achieved when the digit is passively extended to its maximum range.

The nylon thread attached to the leather loop is then threaded through this hole. Rubber bands are attached to the nylon thread at a distance of 5–7 cm from their exit through the outrigger.

These bands are then attached to a hook which is bonded on to the proximal edge of the splint.

Regular review of this splint is necessary so that adjustments to the angle of pull can be made commensurate with improvement of the contracture.

Dorsal finger extension splint

See Figure 6.3a.

Indications

To maintain extension where the IP joints are not resistant to passive extension, e.g.:

1 Mallet finger (splint worn across DIP joint only).
2 To arrest the early tendency to PIP flexion contracture, e.g. following flexor tendon surgery or PIP joint arthroplasty.
3 Buttonhole deformity. The splint is worn across the PIP joint only, allowing DIP flexion.
4 To maintain correction of a PIP joint flexion contracture after removal of a dorsal outrigger.

Materials

1 Ezeform or San-Splint XR.
2 Adhesive foam lining.
3 Non-adhesive Velcro hook.
4 Velcro pile.
5 Adhesive Velcro hook.

Construction

1 The length and width of the digit are measured and the splint cut accordingly.
2 The splint is lined with an adhesive foam which does not have a tendency to 'bottom out'.
3 The dorsum of the splint is covered with adhesive Velcro hook to which one end of each of the Velcro pile straps is attached.
4 The small square of non-adhesive Velcro hook is sewn on to the smooth side at the end of the Velcro pile strap which attaches on to the splint. Each strap is wound around the finger and then attached to itself.

Joint jack

See Figure 10.10.
    This commercial splint provides a steady non-elastic force that is easily controlled by the patient.

Indications

PIP and/or DIP joint flexion deformity of 35 degrees or less which is resistant to passive extension.

Capener splint (spring-wire PIP joint extension splint)

See Figure 5.8.

Indications

1 Flexion deformity of 30–45 degrees which is not strongly resistant to passive extension.
2 Extension splinting for conservative management of a button-hole deformity.

Materials and tools

1 Spring steel piano wire 17 Gauge
2 Jig for turning coils (Figure 15.10) (This jig is available commercially; design specifications for the manufacture of the jig can be found in Wynn Parry (1981) or Barr (1975).
3 Long-nosed pliers.
4 Wire cutters.
5 Moleskin.
6 Orfit (thinnest gauge).

Construction

1 Cut a length of approximately 37 cm of piano wire.

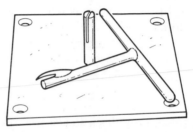

Figure 15.10   *Jig for turning coils*

2 Using the long-nosed pliers to hold the wire, form a U-shape in the wire at its centre, ensuring that the curve formed is a smooth one. The wires should remain parallel and the frame is slightly wider than the width of the finger.

3 Place the U-shape on the volar aspect of the finger with the curve resting at the distal palmar crease; mark the wire with liquid paper just distal to the finger web spaces on the radial and ulnar sides of the finger (Figure 15.11).

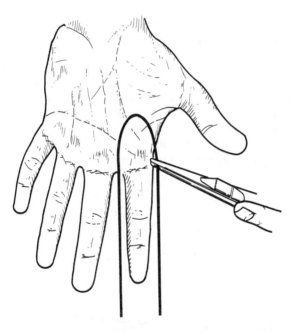

Figure 15.11   *Smooth U-shape is formed at the centre of the wire; this curve rests at the distal palmar crease*

4 Bend the wire on both sides at an angle of 60 degrees so that the wires pass between the fingers; the wires are then bent again at an angle of 60 degrees so that they now lie mid-laterally along the finger. Ensure that the wires remain parallel (Figure 15.12).

5 With the splint placed on the volar aspect of the finger, mark the axis of the PIP joint.

6 This point is then placed in the middle of the slot in the jig.

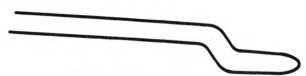

Figure 15.12 *Following the bending of the 60 degree angles, ensure that the wires remain parallel and that they lie mid-laterally along the finger.*

The jig handle is placed over the base and two complete revolutions are turned while a downward pressure on the wire is maintained.

The coil is always turned toward the volar aspect of the digit if an extension force is to be provided. Throughout the manoeuvre it must be ensured that the coil is turned at a right angle to the axis of the parallel wires.

7 The splint is repositioned in the jig and the second coil is turned (Figure 15.13).

8 The base curve of the splint is covered with a double layer of the thinnest gauge Orfit and moulded on to the palm for comfort.

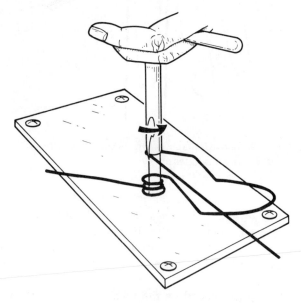

Figure 15.13 *Second coil is turned ensuring that this procedure is performed at a right angle to the axis of the parallel wires*

9 Adhesive moleskin is used to fashion a dorsal hood over the proximal phalanx and a corresponding 'sling' to cradle the underside (or volar aspect) of the middle phalanx.

The width of the dorsal hood extends from the interdigital web space to the PIP joint; the width of the distal 'sling' is the length of the middle phalanx but can be extended over the DIP joint for extra leverage.

The length of the hood and sling should allow the coils to sit in the mid-lateral position of the digit.

10 Using the wire snips, cut off excess wire, leaving a short length which can be turned back on to itself, with the long-nosed pliers, in a tight loop for safety.

Serial plaster casting for PIP joint flexion contracture

See Figure 15.14.

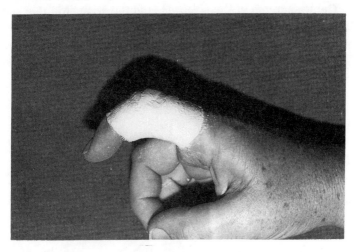

Figure 15.14 *Serial plaster casting of a contracted PIP joint*

Indications

Moderate to severe PIP joint flexion contracture (70–90 degrees) which has been long-standing or where dynamic traction has not been successful.

Materials

1 Strips of plaster bandage approximately 30–37 cm in length.
2 Lanolin to protect the skin.

Method

1 A film of lanolin is smoothed over the area to be covered by the plaster.
2 With the wrist and MCP joints relaxed in a slightly flexed position, e.g. over the edge of a table, the plaster strip is applied in a proximal to distal direction from the web space to just short of the DIP joint.

   Throughout this manoeuvre and while the cast is setting, a gentle stretch of the PIP joint into extension is maintained. Two overlapping wraps of plaster are usually sufficient to make a firm cast.
3 The cast is removed after 2–3 days and the hand washed.

   Gentle active exercises are carried out to ensure that flexion range is not lost.

   A new cast is then applied in the corrected position. This procedure is repeated every few days until it is deemed that no further gains are likely to be made.

Thumb rotation strap

See Figure 4.9.

Indication

Median nerve palsy with inability to rotate and oppose the thumb to the index finger.

Materials

1 Leather or neoprene for wrist strap.
2 Velcro hook and pile.
3 Velfoam strap approximately 24 × 4 cm.
4 Possibly foam lining for extra comfort to the wrist strap.

Construction

1 The circumference of the wrist is measured, allowing for a 4 cm overlap for Velcro closure. The width of the wrist strap is approximately 5 cm.
2 A 3 cm wide strip of non-adhesive Velcro hook is machine-sewn on to the outside of the wrist strap, extending along its entire length. For extra comfort and to minimize movement of the strap at the wrist, it is lined with an adhesive-backed foam such as Polycushion or Kushionflex.
3 One end of the Velfoam strap is attached to the wrist strap just below the CMC joint of the thumb. The ˙strap is looped anteriorly around the thenar eminence and across the dorsum of the MCP joint; it is then drawn obliquely across the hand to attach to the wrist strap over the distal end of the ulna. The ends of the strap are tapered to 2 cm for neatness and ease of attachment.

The tension of the strap is such that opposition is maintained without undue tightness.

C-splint

See Figures 2.14 and 10.12.

Indication

Where there is reduction in thumb web span following:

1 Peripheral nerve lesion.
2 Tendon or nerve repair to the thumb.
3 Any injury requiring lengthy immobilization.

Materials

1 Ezeform.
2 5 cm bandage to hold the splint in position.

Construction

1 Several minutes are spent gently stretching the thumb web to accommodate the splint in a slightly corrected position. It must be ensured that the stretch is occurring in the actual web space and not at the thumb IP joint.

2 A tape measure is laid along the arc extending from the tip of the index finger to just beyond the tip of the thumb and this distance is measured.

The width of the splint is usually 4–5 cm depending on the size of the hand. If the splint is too narrow, it will not fit comfortably and has a tendency to shift.

3 The heated material is moulded into the web space and held in the corrected position until the material has hardened.

C-splints are used serially; the splint can be re-heated a number of times and may need to be renewed before the maximum web span is obtained.

Thumb post (hand-based)

See Figures 5.13, 13.4 and 15.15.

Indications

1 Protection and immobilization following injury to or repair of the ulnar collateral ligament of the MCP joint of the thumb.
2 Support to the first CMC joint with osteoarthritis.

Materials

1 Orfit (thinnest gauge) or San-Splint XR.
2 2.5 cm elasticated Velcro pile.

Construction

1 The softened material is placed around the thumb where it is 'pinched' together inside the web space. Any excess material is carefully cut away with the splinting shears.
2 Splint is effectively secured with the 2.5 cm elasticated Velcro which is attached in a cross-over fashion on the volar aspect of the splint at the level of the first CMC joint.

Thumb post (forearm-based)

See Figure 5.15.

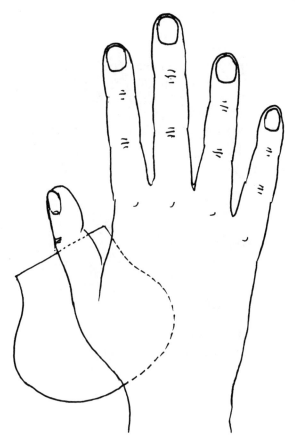

Figure 15.15   *Pattern for a hand-based thumb post used to immobilize the first CMC joint and MCP joint of the thumb*

Indications

1 Immobilization following trapezium arthroplasty.
2 Support in the management of De Quervain's syndrome (stenosing tenosynovitis of EPB and APL in the first dorsal compartment).
3 As a basis for a dynamic low-profile IP joint flexion splint (Figure 15.16).

The pattern for the forearm-based thumb post is simply an extension of the thumb post for the hand.

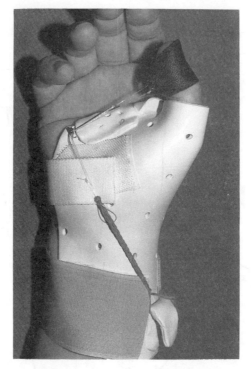

Figure 15.16   *Dynamic low-profile flexion splint for the IP joint of the thumb*

To make a low-profile dynamic IP joint flexion splint, follow the guidelines describing manufacture of the low-profile MCP joint flexion splint mentioned earlier in this chapter.

Low-profile dynamic flexion splint for thumb MCP joint

See Figures 15.17 and 15.18.

Indication

Stiffness of the MCP joint following injury or surgery.

The pattern for this splint is a short version of a gauntlet-type cock-up splint.

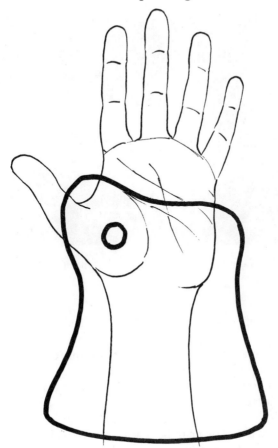

Figure 15.17 *Pattern of gauntlet-type cock-up splint which can be used as the basis for a low-profile dynamic flexion splint for the thumb MCP joint*

For the making of this splint, follow the guidelines describing manufacture of the low-profile MCP joint flexion splint.

Lycra fingerstalls

See Figure 2.16.

Lycra is a two-way stretch material made from nylon and elastic. The stretch in Lycra is not equal in both directions and

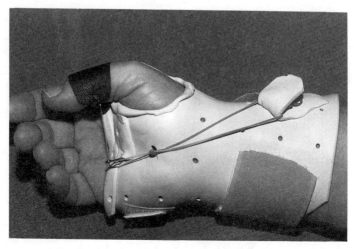

Figure 15.18 *Low-profile dynamic flexion splint for the thumb MCP joint*

the degree of stretch and texture varies between different materials.

Lycra fingerstalls are an effective means of treating digital oedema and digital scarring.

They are contraindicated where oedema is a result of inflammation or infection.

Fingerstalls can be fitted as soon as sutures are removed and the wound is dry. They can be worn continuously, being removed for bathing and laundering.

Exercises and activities can be performed with the stall in place and splints can be applied over the stall.

Fingerstalls should be reviewed regularly and their tension adjusted as oedema and scarring resolve.

Manufacture

See Figure 15.19.

The garment should be cut with maximum stretch in a proximal-distal direction, the gradient of pressure being increased in the same direction.

If oedema is confined to the PIP joint, the finger tip can remain free, ensuring that the distal edge of the stall is 'baggy' so as not to compromise the circulation.

Index or middle fingers   Ring or little fingers

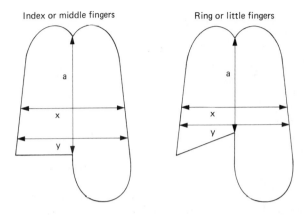

Figure 15.19 *Pattern for Lycra fingerstall. Measurements: a, distance from tip of digit to interdigital web, minus approximately 0.5 cm to allow for stretch; x, circumference of PIP joint plus 0.5 cm for seam; y, circumference of proximal phalanx plus 0.5 cm for seam*

Tension of the stall should be sufficient to be perceived as gentle compression by the patient; however, it should not result in throbbing, numbness or discoloration of the digit.

The pattern for the fingerstall is drafted from circumferential and linear measurements.

A slight modification is necessary when drafting stalls for the ring and little fingers to allow for the natural slant at the bases of these digits.

References and further reading

Barr, N. R. (1975) *The Hand: Principles and Techniques of Simple Splintmaking in Rehabilitation*, Butterworths, London, pp. 79–80

Baillière's Nurses' Dictionary, 17th edition (1968), Baillière Tindall, London

Brand, P. (1990) The forces of dynamic splinting: ten questions before applying a dynamic splint to the hand. In *Rehabilitation of the Hand: Surgery and Therapy*, 3rd edn. (eds J. M. Hunter, L. H. Schneider, E. J. Mackin *et al.*), C. V. Mosby, St Louis, pp. 1095–1100

Colditz, J. C. (1983) Low profile dynamic splinting of the injured hand. *American Journal of Occupational Therapy*, **37**, 182–188

English, C. B., Rehm, R. A. and Petzoldt, R. L. (1982) Blocking splints to assist finger exercises. *American Journal of Occupational Therapy*, **36**, 259–262

Fess, E. E. and Philips, C. A. (1987) *Hand Splinting: Principles and Methods*, 2nd edn, C. V. Mosby, St. Louis

Gribben, M. G. (1986) Splinting principles for hand injuries. In *Hand Rehabilitation* (ed. C. A. Moran) Churchill Livingstone, New York, pp. 159–189

Hunter, J. M., Schneider, L. H., Mackin, E.J. *et al.* (eds) (1990) Splinting. In *Rehabilitation of the Hand: Surgery and Therapy* 3rd edn, C. V. Mosby, St Louis, pp. 1095–1152

Kiel, J. (1983) *Basic Hand Splinting: a Pattern-Designing Approach*, Little, Brown, Boston

Malick, M. H. (1976) *Manual on Static Hand Splinting*, 3rd edn, Harmarville Rehabilitation Centre, Pittsburgh

Malick, M. H. (1978) *Manual on Dynamic Hand Splinting with Thermoplastic Materials*, 2nd edn, Harmarville Rehabilitation Centre, Pittsburgh

Moberg, E. (1984) *Splinting in Hand Therapy*, Thieme-Stratton, New York

Morrin, J., Taylor, K. and Conolly, W. B. (1981) Control of hand oedema by the use of Lycra pressure garments. *Australian Occupational Therapy Journal*, **28**, 167–174

Wynn Parry, C. B. (1981) *Rehabilitation of the Hand*, 4th edn, Butterworth, London, pp. 75–77

Ziegler, E. M. (ed.) (1984) *Current Concepts in Orthotics: A diagnosis Related Approach to Splinting*, Rolyan Medical Products, USA

List of suppliers

Australian

Total Patient Care
17 Windsor Road
Northmead NSW 2152
Tel: 6835360, 6835363.

Smith and Nephew Pty. Ltd
4 Bessemer Street
Blacktown NSW 2148
Tel: 6713100

Vikora Pty. Ltd
95 O'Sullivan Road
Rose Bay, NSW 2029
Tel: 3277609

Boehringer Mannheim Pty. Ltd
31 Victoria Avenue
Castle Hill, NSW 2154
Tel: 8997999

Dow Corning Pty. Ltd
4 Ray Road,
Epping, NSW 2121
Tel: 8689111

Johnson and Johnson
154 Pacific Highway
St. Leonards, NSW 2065
Tel: 4390066

UK and Europe

Beiersdorf Ltd
Yeomans Drive
Blakelands
Milton Keynes MK14 5LS
Tel: 0908 211444, Fax: 0908 211555

Bissell Healthcare Ltd
Northgate House
Staple Gardens
Winchester SO23 8ST

Centromed Ltd
Fairwood Industrial Park
Stafford Close
Ashford TN23 2TT

Chattanooga Group Inc.
Goods Road
Belpher
Derbyshire

DTR Medical
220 Cathays Terrace
Cardiff CF1 4JA

Hugh Steeper Ltd
Queen Mary's University Hospital
Roehampton Lane
London SW15 5PL

Huntleigh Healthcare
310–312 Dallow Road
Luton LU1 1SS

Nottingham Rehabilitation Ltd
Ludlow Hill Road
West Bridgford
Nottingham NG2 6HD

3M Healthcare Ltd (see 3M Riker)
3M Riker
Morley Street
Loughborough LE11 1EP
Tel: 0509 611611

Johnson and Johnson Patient Care Ltd
Coronation Road
Ascot S15 9EY
Tel: 0990 872626

Smith and Nephew Ltd
PO Box 81
101 Hessle Road
Hull HU3 2BN
Tel: 0482 25181

Smith and Nephew Pharmaceuticals
Bampton Road
Harold Hill
Romford RM3 8SL
Tel: 04023 49333

Dynasplint Systems Inc.
De Koumen 82
6433 KE Heerlen
The Netherlands

Enraf Nonius Delft
PO Box 810
2600 AV Delft
The Netherlands

Kebo Care AS
Jerikoveion 28
Postboks 1
Leirdal
1008 Oslo 1
Norway

USA

North Coast Medical Inc.
187 Stauffer Boulevard,
San Jose,
CA 95125-1042
Tel: 408 283 1900
Fax: 408 283 1950

Fred Sammons Inc. (A Bissell Healthcare Company)
PO Box 3697 Dept 910
Grand Rapids MI 49501 3697

AliMed Inc.
297 High Street
Dedham, MA 02026
Tel: 800 225 2610
In MA Tel: 617 329 2900

Smith and Nephew Rolyan, Inc.
Tel: 1 800 558 8633

The Joint-Jack Company
108 Britt Road
East Hartford, CT 06118
Tel: 203 568 7338

Jamar (Hand Dynamometers)
Tel: 800 527 7530
In NJ Tel: 201 777 8004

Index